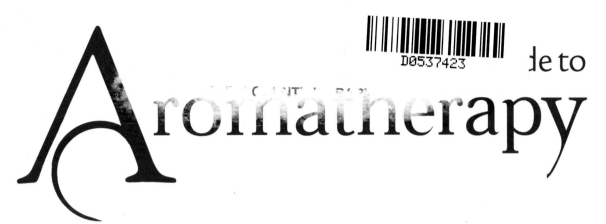

de to

Aromatherapy

Louise Tucker

General Editor Jane Foulston

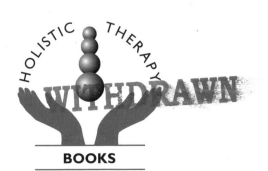

HOLISTIC THERAPY

BOOKS

Published by Holistic Therapy Books
An imprint of Ruben Publishing Ltd.
P.O. Box 270
Cambridge
CB1 2XE
Tel: 01223 500344

First published November 2000.
Revised July 2004.

ISBN 1-903348-01-3.

Set in 10/13 Legacy.

Printed by Scotprint, Haddington.

Prepared for the publishers by The Write Idea, Cambridge.

Contents

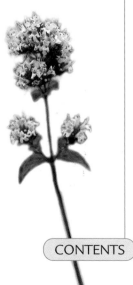

Introduction

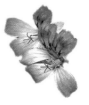

This book provides a clearly explained and illustrated introduction to aromatherapy. Ideal for students and professionals, it covers everything from the history of essential oils to their present-day uses and applications.

Author

Louise Tucker

Louise Tucker is a freelance writer. Previously an academic and tutor, she has written books on various subjects, including *An Introductory Guide to Anatomy and Physiology*, also published by Holistic Therapy Books.

General Editor

Jane Foulston

Jane Foulston has had a long career as a lecturer in anatomy and physiology for beauty and complementary therapy in private and FE colleges as well as setting up a school in Japan. She also has 15 years' experience as an external examiner for professional vocational qualifications. She lectured at East Berkshire College and Bridgewater College and her students have become practitioners in beauty therapy, aromatherapy and in a variety of sports therapies. She is currently Director of the International Therapy Examination Council.

Contributing Editors

Fae Major

Fae Major has worked in the beauty therapy industry for 23 years. She qualified with international diplomas in 1981, and her work has included three years working for Steiners International Hair and Beauty, one year in an alternative medicine clinic, two years in a small private salon in the north of England and a short spell in a salon in Barbados. For the last 16 years she has been teaching beauty therapy and aromatherapy, and in 1992 she became a practical examiner for ITEC, and has been a theory examination marker since 2002.

Marguerite Wynne

Marguerite Wynne began her career in one of London's foremost beauty salons and went on to teach in The College of Beauty Therapy in the West End. Subsequently, she owned her own clinic and school in Buckinghamshire, specialising in Complementary Therapies. She has been a Chief Examiner for ITEC since 1985 during which time she has spent three years based in the Far East.

Elaine Hall

Elaine Hall began her career teaching beauty and complementary therapies at the West of England College in Bath. She then went on to manage the complementary therapies section at Bridgwater College. Since then Elaine has run her own private salon and clinic based within a nursing home where she has treated both the elderly and private clients. In addition she has held the post of Senior ITEC Examiner and she examines extensively both in the South West of England and overseas.

Acknowledgements

The publishers would like to thank the following for their invaluable assistance in the preparation of this book:

Louise Barnes ITEC qualified Aromatherapist and Beauty Therapist
Louise Oakley Model
Claire Bowman BA Hons Photography
Elaine Hall Senior Examiner ITEC
Fae Major Senior Examiner ITEC
Marguerite Wynne Chief Examiner ITEC
Cariad Supplier of essential oils for the photographs

We would also like to acknowledge the assistance of the following photographic agencies for supplying many of the images used:
Heather Angel
A–Z Botanical Collection Ltd
Harry Smith Horticultural Photographic Collection
Garden Matters
John Fielding Slide Library

1 The history and origins of aromatherapy

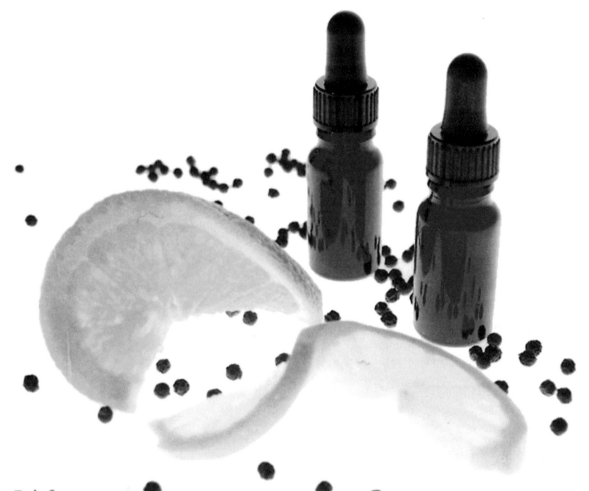

In Brief

Aromatherapy is the use of essential oils from plants for their therapeutic properties. The oils are used for treating medical and non-medical conditions. Although it may appear to be a relatively new therapy, plant oils have been used for their health benefits for centuries.

Learning objectives

The target knowledge of this chapter is:
● the history of aromatherapy
● the development of aromatherapy
● the definition of aromatherapy.

HISTORY

What is aromatherapy?

Aromatherapy is the systematic use of essential oils in holistic treatments to improve physical and emotional well-being. Essential oils, extracted from plants, possess distinctive therapeutic properties which can be used to improve health and prevent disease. Both their physiological and psychological effects combine well to promote positive health. These natural plant oils are applied in a variety of ways including massage, baths and inhalations.

An Egyptian tomb.

They are readily absorbed into the skin and have gentle physiological effects. Aromatherapy is an especially effective treatment for stress-related problems and a variety of chronic conditions. The name dates from the 1920s but different cultures and civilisations, such as the Ancient Egyptians and the Roman Empire, have used plants and herbs for religious, medical and cosmetic purposes, as well as in rituals, embalming and preserving, for centuries.

'The Cradle of Medicine'

The Egyptians are known to have used plant resins and essences in preserving the dead. Cedar and myrrh were used in embalming and jars of frankincense and styrax have been found by archaeologists in tombs dating from 3000BC. The antiseptic and antibacterial qualities of the oils and essences helped to prevent dead bodies from rotting so that, when mummies were discovered thousands of years later, they were perfectly preserved. In a hot country with little sanitation, plant extracts and oils made life more pleasant! Some of the prescriptions and formulae were inscribed onto stone tablets which is one of the reasons we know so much about them today.

The Greeks

The Nile Valley in Egypt was known as the 'Cradle of Medicine' and other cultures, especially the ancient Greeks gained much of their knowledge from travelling to this area and taking the information home.

Hippocrates (born around 460BC) was a Greek and he was an important person in the development of the use of plants in medicine. He also wrote on the subject, thus helping others to understand the useful properties of plants and herbs.

The Arab influence

Any history of aromatherapy should mention a Persian called Abd Allah ibn Sina (980–1037), usually referred to as Avicenna, who contributed a great deal to medicine both past and present. Firstly, he described accurately about eight hundred plants and their uses. Secondly, he devised very detailed instructions on massage and thirdly, he is credited with discovering the process of distillation by which most of our essential oils are obtained.

An Egyptian mummy.

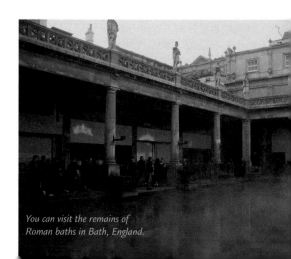

You can visit the remains of Roman baths in Bath, England.

The first scented baths?

The Romans had a huge Empire, which existed for over 500 years (from 27BC until around the fifth century AD). They had conquered many other countries and had access to all the plants and oils of those countries. Oils and essences were an important part of Roman culture. For example, they were used at the public baths, in the water and in massage. This might not seem very significant to us, but baths were a central part of a Roman's daily life. They were like present-day cafés and pubs: this was where you went not only to get a wash and massage but also to chat to friends, family and business associates.

Four millennia of experience

China and India both have a long history of using plants and herbs and their extracts for medical purposes. In India medicine is aimed at healing the whole body i.e. treating physical, spiritual and psychological problems all at the same time. Traditional Indian herbal medicine, known as Ayurvedic medicine, dates from thousands of years ago as does Chinese medicine. Now, in 2000AD, 4000 years later, the use of Chinese medical treatments such as acupuncture, shiatsu or herbal remedies is becoming widespread.

From the Crusades to the Great Plague: Europe's role

Europe learnt about the health benefits of plants and herbs through the travels of knights and soldiers who brought back news of their use, especially after the Crusades (from the eleventh to the thirteenth century). Gradually, Europeans began to experiment with herbal remedies made from plants and herbs that grew in their own countries, like sage, lavender and rosemary. In the Middle Ages people protected themselves against infection by carrying

> **Did you know?**
>
> Frankincense means pure incense, from the Old French 'franc encens'. Though we might think that frankincense and myrrh are poor gifts compared to gold, we are using modern values to compare them. The fact that they were presented at an important event such as the birth of Jesus suggests that they were worth just as much if not more than gold. Frankincense is still used as part of the incense burned in some churches. See Adrian Room (Ed), *Brewer's Dictionary of Phrase and Fable*, p. 420.

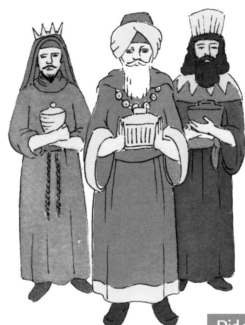

In the Bible, the three kings brought gifts to baby Jesus, including frankincense and myrrh.

plants, wearing herbal bouquets and throwing both over the floor. During the Great Plague perfumers and apothecaries were thought to be immune from the disease. Using flowers and plants against germs might sound superstitious but think of how many lavender, pine and sandalwood disinfectants and cleaning products we now have in our lives! And gipsies still sell lucky bunches of herbs to ward off evil.

Blinding with science

The development of chemistry and printing in the nineteenth century helped

> **Did you know?**
>
> That during the Roman Empire, essences and resins were so expensive that slaves who worked at the baths were checked by security before they went home to make sure they hadn't stolen any valuable essences!

> **Did you know?**
>
> In China, the Yellow Emperor's Book of Internal Medicine is one of the earliest records of the use of herbal medicine, dating back to at least 2000 years BC. See Julia Lawless, *The Encyclopaedia of Essential Oils*, p. 12.

herbal and plant medicine in two ways. New chemical processes made it easier to extract oils and the invention of printing meant that lots of books on the subject, called herbals, were published. However, science helped both to develop the use of plants and herbs in medicines and to destroy it. It became easier and cheaper to discover some of the elements of plant oils, and their qualities, and attempt to produce synthetic versions of them. So commercial, mass-produced products and remedies using artificial ingredients replaced the natural formulas created for the individual person and problem. Herbal medicine, using ancient and tested traditions was no longer taken seriously and was even considered 'quackery' compared to 'real' scientific medicine.

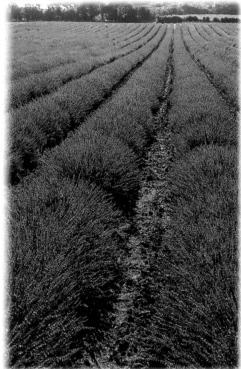

A field of lavender.

The 'invention' of aromatherapy

The term aromatherapy was coined by a French chemist called René Maurice Gattefossé in the 1920s. He was a chemist and perfumier who worked in his family perfumery business. One day he burnt his hand and plunged it into a vat of lavender oil to cool it down. He discovered that the lavender oil helped his burns to heal and prevented scarring. During the First World War (1914-1918) he used oils on soldiers' wounds and discovered that they helped heal wounds much faster. He went on to research the therapeutic properties of essential oils

and first used the phrase *aromathérapie* in a scientific research paper he delivered in 1928. Several other French scientists, including Dr Jean Valnet, continued the research into the effect of essential oils on physical burns and wounds as well as psychological disorders. Valnet also used oils on soldiers' wounds, this time during the Second World War (1939-1945), because of their antiseptic qualities.

Aromatherapy reaches Britain

Marguerite Maury, an Austrian biochemist and follower of the work of Valnet, is the person responsible for bringing aromatherapy to Britain. She had discovered that when she used essential oils in massage the skin absorbed the oils very well. In the 1940s she brought her ideas for massage treatments using essential oils to this country and, with the help of several people (including Micheline Arcier, Dr W. E. Arnould-Taylor, Eve Taylor and Dr Jean Valnet) she set up aromatherapy practices. Her students then set up their own practices and the interest in this method of treatment has been growing ever since. Furthermore, although first established as a beauty therapy, aromatherapy was developed as a clinical (i.e. medical) therapy by Robert Tisserand.

Full circle

Thanks to Gattefossé and his followers, aromatherapy began to be taken seriously again. The reputation of complementary therapies is now coming full circle. A move away from orthodox medicine and commercial drugs has coincided with, or perhaps caused a surge of interest in the use of natural complementary therapies. Traditional medicine now uses more and more such therapies to complement treatments of physical and psychological conditions.

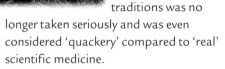

2 Essential oils and where they come from

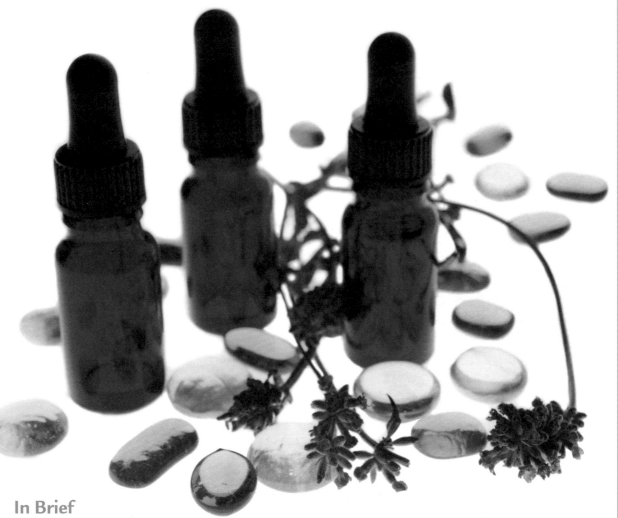

In Brief

In order to understand the present-day use of plant and herb oils in aromatherapy and other treatments, we need to learn exactly what an essential oil is. The following section provides a definition and description of essential oils as well as explaining the different methods for extracting them from plants.

Learning objectives

The target knowledge of this chapter is:
- the definition of essential oils
- extraction methods
- the importance of using quality oils
- synergy
- chemotypes.

WHAT ARE ESSENTIAL OILS?

Essential oils are aromatic, volatile substances extracted from a single botanical source by distillation or expression. They are found in leaves, the hairs on leaves, in flowers, in tree bark or roots, in fruit pulp and peel. Similar to animal hormones, they are sometimes referred to as the plants' 'life force'. Generally, the cells containing them are close to the surface but they can only be seen with the help of a microscope, not just by looking at a leaf or flower. The essence is either stored in the cell where it is made or, as is the case with citrus fruits, moved to special storage sacs.

Essential oils are:

- aromatic – have a distinctive and often fragrant smell
- volatile – evaporate quickly in the air and to varying degrees depending on the oil
- very powerful when neat – are usually blended with a carrier oil for massage purposes (see Chapter 4)
- flammable – must be kept in a cool place away from heat and/or naked flames
- soluble in oil and alcohol (in water they will form a suspension i.e. particles of the oil can be suspended in the water but will not mix with it)
- liquid – exceptions include rose otto and benzoin which are semi-solid
- non-greasy – despite their name, the oils are generally light and not oily!
- expensive – producing the plants and extracting the oil is labour intensive and thus not cheap.

You now know what an essential oil is. The next section explains how they are extracted: how they get from the plant to the bottle!

WHERE DO THEY COME FROM?

A NOTE ON PRICE

The price of an oil reflects two main factors: the time and energy required to produce and harvest the plants and the weight of material or number of flowers required to produce a certain amount of oil. Since there is more oil contained in a leaf than in a petal, oils from leaves will be cheaper than oils from flowers. So sage, thyme and rosemary, from leaves, will be cheaper than jasmine or rose which come from petals. This means that the amount of raw material required to produce different oils varies enormously: whereas only 400kg of thyme will produce 1kg of essential thyme oil, 2000kg of rose petals are needed to produce 1kg of rose oil. And to obtain just 1kg of jasmine oil, one of the most expensive available, four million jasmine flowers are needed...and, since they can only be harvested by hand, in the afternoon and evening, the production process is very expensive!

Essential oils come from various parts of the plants. Some plants only produce one oil e.g.

- basil oil – from basil leaves
- carrot – from carrot seeds
- pine – from the needles and sometimes the cones of pine trees.

Other plants produce several oils from different parts. For example, the orange tree can produce three essential oils:

- petitgrain – from the leaves and branches
- neroli – from the blossom
- orange – from the peel of the fruit.

EXTRACTION METHODS

How do the oils get from the plant to the bottle?

The first stage of production is growing the plants! This process, like every other process in the essential oil industry is labour intensive and therefore expensive. This is because the plants must be looked after very carefully, sometimes by hand (to prevent machinery causing damage and wasting the oil). Once harvested, the plants need to be processed in order to extract the essential oils. There are seven methods of extraction:

- steam distillation
- expression
- solvent extraction
- carbon dioxide extraction
- hydro-diffusion/percolation
- enfleurage
- maceration (an old method which is rarely used today).

Steam distillation

This is the most common and economical method of extraction. Plant material is placed in the first part of a still (see diagram). It is either mixed with water which is then heated to produce steam or steam under pressure is passed through the plant material. The heat and steam cause the essential oil in the plant material to break down and evaporate into the steam. The mix of steam and oil vapour passes into a cooled pipe and condenses (turns back into liquid). The now-liquid mix passes into a collecting vessel where the oil and water, which are of different densities, separate making it easy to decant the oil. There are five stages to distillation:

1. **plant preparation**: flowers and leaves and any non-woody or fibrous parts of plants can be put in the still as they are. But if the oil is from a wood (like sandalwood or rosewood) or a seed (like carrot seed) then the raw material needs to be prepared. Woody parts, like branches or twigs must be grated; anything with a husk or shell (seeds) must be crushed and fruits must be cut. This is necessary to break the walls of the plants' oil cells and release the oil.

2. **heat**: in steam distillation the raw material (leaves, petals, wood etc) is placed on a grid over water which is then heated and steam passed through the plant; in direct distillation the raw material is placed in water which is then brought to boiling point.

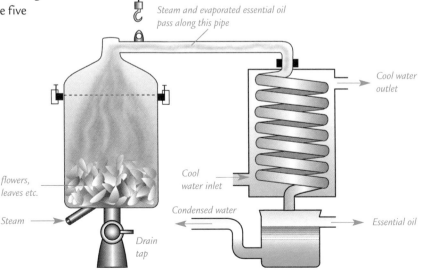

Distillation plant.

Steam and evaporated essential oil pass along this pipe

Cool water outlet

Cool water inlet

Condensed water

Essential oil

flowers, leaves etc.

Steam

Drain tap

● Did you know?

Have you ever wondered why windows steam up, especially in winter? This is condensation. The warm air indoors comes into contact with the glass of the window, which is much colder, and droplets of water in the air condense, leaving you with steamed-up windows.

3. **evaporation**: the heat makes the oil cells release their essence and the oil evaporates into the steam.

● Did you know?

Have you ever noticed that when you peel an orange your hands become covered in an orange substance? Or that if you are not careful the peel squirts liquid into your eyes? This liquid is the orange's essential oil and it is contained in the 'pores' of the peel: tiny sacs under the surface that give the peel its bumpy/dotty appearance.

4. **condensation**: the steam and the vapour it contains collect in a pipe and are transported to a condenser (a coiled pipe which is immersed in a tank of cold water). As soon as the hot steam and vapour come into contact with the cold pipe, they begin to condense i.e. they turn back into liquids.

5. **collection**: the steam condenses and becomes very lightly scented water, (known as aromatic waters or hydrolats) whereas the plant's oil, which is not the same density as water floats to the top of the 'liquefied steam' or sinks to the bottom (depending on the oil). The essential oil can now be collected.

A solvent extractor.

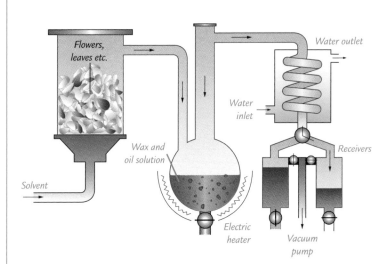

Flowers, leaves etc.

Water outlet

Water inlet

Wax and oil solution

Receivers

Solvent

Electric heater

Vacuum pump

NB The heat used in steam distillation may alter some of the essential oil molecules. Thus the evacuated steam distillation method is sometimes used commercially to avoid this problem. This involves taking as much air as possible out of the distilling equipment (hence 'evacuated') which reduces the air pressure inside. The water used to create the steam therefore boils at a lower temperature which lessens the damage to the oil.

Expression

The oils of citrus fruits (e.g. orange, lemon, grapefruit, mandarin and bergamot) are contained in tiny sacs in the peel. These oils are extracted by the application of pressure. The fruit's pulp and pith are removed and the peel is squeezed to release its oil. Expression used to be done by hand (the oil was collected on sponges) but now, due to the enormous demand for essential oils, machines are used.

NB Strictly speaking, expression extracts the plant's pure essence rather than its essential oil, since the oil obtained is exactly the same as that contained in the plant whereas essential oils are not exactly the same composition as the essence because they have come into contact with other substances, like water or solvents, or been heated. Any oil extracted by a cold, pressed method (i.e. one that simply uses pressure and no heat) is a true essence. This is a bit like olive oil: extra virgin olive oil, i.e. the best and purest, is cold-pressed because the olives have simply been crushed, no heat has been used and no change in composition has taken place.

Solvent extraction

Solvent extraction is the method used when the aromatic essence is difficult to obtain by distillation (e.g. resinoids) or when the process of distillation might damage the delicate fragrance of the plant (e.g. rose and jasmine). There are three types:

● **resinoid e.g. benzoin, myrrh**
When the bark of a tree or a bush is

cut it seems to bleed: a liquid escapes from the cut which solidifies when it comes into contact with air. This semi-solid substance is known as a resin or gum. The aromatic essence of these resins is difficult to obtain through distillation because they are often mixed up with tough fibrous material such as bark and dirt. There are three stages for extracting a resinoid:

1. *preparation*: the raw material is chopped and cut, then placed on a rack in a clean vessel and covered with solvents such as hydrocarbons (e.g. benzene or hexane) or alcohols.

2. *heat*: the mixture is gently heated and the oils contained in the woody plant material dissolve in the solvent.

3. *filtration*: the solvent is evaporated off and the solid residue is called a resinoid.

- **concrete**
When a plant's essential oil is damaged by the hot water or steam used in distillation (for example the fragrance of jasmine flowers is affected by water), solvent extraction is used instead to obtain a solid substance called a concrete, a mixture of natural waxes and a plant's aromatic essence. They are highly concentrated and more 'stable' (i.e they do not evaporate when exposed to the air) than pure essential oils. Similar to resin extraction, this process uses hydrocarbon solvents and has three stages:

1. *preparation*: the raw material is put on racks in clean sealed vessels and covered with solvent.

2. *heat*: the mixture is gently heated and the solvent dissolves the essences contained in the plant material.

3. *filtration*: the liquid that remains is filtered to remove the solvent. The semi-solid paste that remains is the concrete.

- **absolutes e.g. rose, jasmine**
After extraction concretes are usually treated further to obtain what is known as an absolute. Absolutes are obtained by mixing a concrete (or a pomade from enfleurage – see below) with alcohol. The aromatic plant essence transfers from the solid waxy substance to the alcohol and the wax which is not soluble in alcohol is left as residue. This process has two stages:

1. *mixing*: the concrete is mixed with alcohol and then chilled. The plant essence in the concrete dissolves in the alcohol and a waxy residue remains.

2. *filtration*: the solution is filtered to separate the waxy residue from the liquid. Then the alcohol is evaporated off, leaving the absolute, the plant's essence.

What is an absolute?
A liquid which is thicker and more highly concentrated than a pure essential oil. Some are solids or semi-solid such as rose absolute, which may solidify at room temperature but turns into a liquid when it gets warmer. Absolutes are generally used in small amounts not only because they are so highly concentrated but also because they may still contain a residue of the extraction solvent and this can cause reactions.

Carbon dioxide extraction
This is quite a new process that dates from the 1980s. It is similar to solvent extraction, in that plant material is brought into contact with a chemical substance, in this case, compressed carbon dioxide (CO_2) at a low temperature. The process is quite complicated and therefore expensive.

Enfleurage

This is an old extraction process that produces a waxy substance, similar to a concrete, known as a pomade. It is very labour-intensive and therefore expensive

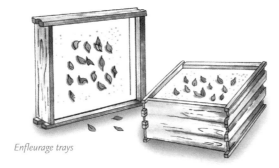

Enfleurage trays

and is rarely used except when the very highest quality oil is required. It only works with flowers which carry on producing essential oils after they have been harvested. The process involves four stages:

1. **extraction**: flowers and petals are placed on trays which have been coated with animal fat. They are left on the trays for several days and the fat absorbs the plant essence. Faded petals are replaced with fresh ones until the fat is completely saturated with the essence.

2. **collection**: the fat is removed from the trays and any remaining petals taken out. The 'aromatic fat' is now known as a pomade.

3. **separation**: the pomade is mixed in alcohol and agitated constantly for a day (this part is carried out by a machine) so that the essential oil can separate from the fat. The fat is removed.

4. **evaporation**: the alcohol is evaporated off from the mixture leaving the enfleurage absolute.

Like other absolutes, those from enfleurage are highly concentrated and are either thick liquids or solids.

Maceration

Maceration is a process similar to enfleurage by which plant material is placed in liquid fixed oils or fat and then heated to 60–70°C. The mixture is stirred and the heat causes the cells containing essential oils to break down, allowing the constituents to be absorbed by the oil or fat. The plant material is then removed and the process repeated until the fixed oil or fat is saturated. The strained plant material is wrapped in bags and cold pressed to obtain any remaining liquid. If fat is used it is called a pomade and can be treated with alcohol as above to produce an absolute.

Infusion

This is a simple method of essential oil extraction that can be used at home with herbs from the garden to make pleasantly scented massage oil. Plant material is placed in a fixed oil and left in a warm place. The essential oils are gradually absorbed by the fixed oils and the plant material is separated. This process can be repeated until the desired concentration is achieved. Calendula is an example of an infused oil.

Hydro-diffusion/Percolation

Percolation uses boiling water in a similar way to distillation but the water passes down through the plant material instead of up. When cooled the oil either floats or sinks, depending on the density and is easily separated. Percolation's main advantage is that it is faster than distillation, which results in less damage to the oil because the essence is heated for a shorter period of time.

You now know where essential oils come from and how they are extracted. The final section in this chapter explains the factors that affect oil quality, some of the different uses of oils and the benefits of using good quality oils.

THE QUALITY OF ESSENTIAL OILS

The previous section explained how essential oils and essences are extracted from all sorts of plants. Production and extraction, as you can see, are time-consuming, laborious and costly which makes the oils very expensive. This, combined with increased demand for essential oils, has created a market for cheaper, poorer quality, artificial or synthetic oils and diluted versions. The next section explains how and why companies and individuals 'adulterate' oils and why oil quality is so important in aromatherapy.

What is adulteration?

Both companies and individuals may adulterate (i.e. change) an expensive pure oil to make it go further and, in some cases make more money. Essential oils can be adulterated as follows:

1. **dilution**: the essential oil is diluted in an alcohol or spirit base. The true aroma is maintained but the product has no therapeutic value e.g. perfume or pot pourri oils.

2. **stretching**: the expensive essential oil may be made to go further by mixing it with a cheaper one or by mixing it with an artificial product that has no colour or smell e.g. petitgrain mixed with the more expensive neroli. Both come from different parts of an orange.

3. **isolation**: a chemical from a cheaper oil may be isolated, removed and mixed with the expensive oil to make it go further e.g. a chemical from lemongrass, which is relatively cheap, is mixed with the very expensive melissa oil.

4. **substitution**: a cheaper oil may be used instead e.g. amyris may be substituted for sandalwood.

It is difficult not only to know the contents of these diluted and adulterated blends but also to detect the synthetic versions. A qualified aromatherapist will always use a reputable supplier, especially since an adulterated oil may not work effectively in treatment.

Why is it important to use real, unadulterated oils?

Because artificial and synthetic oils and the diluted versions do not have the same therapeutic effects. It is the plant's essence, not a copy of its essence or a tenth of its essence mixed with another oil, which has healing qualities. Egyptian mummies are unlikely to have been so well-preserved if they had been embalmed with adulterated plant essences! The pure oil is made up of hundreds of different chemical constituents, many of which are still unknown to scientists, and mixed together they produce a particular synergy, and this synergistic force and blend cannot be copied by a synthetic substance.

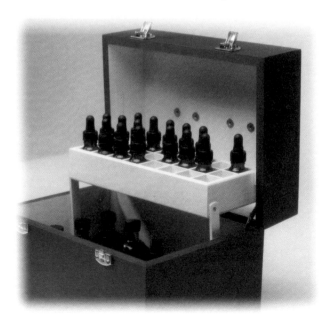

Essential oils are stored out of the light, as in this box.

What is synergy?

The word synergy comes from Greek: the syn comes from the Greek sun, meaning with or together; ergy comes from the greek ergon to work i.e. to work together. Synergy or a synergistic effect in aromatherapy means that when two or more oils work together they produce more of an effect than they do alone. Research has been done on the individual chemical constituents of essential oils and their qualities and effects; what isn't known is how they work together and/or produce effects that are not expected given their chemical make-up and what is known about them.

Can anyone benefit from using synthetics?

Yes, industry. Perfume, pharmaceutical and food industries use essential oils to give their products pleasant smells and flavours e.g. peppermint is used in toothpaste and chewing gum. They need standard smells, not those that are subject to environmental change caused by temperature, storage conditions and where the plant was cultivated. For their purposes synthetic fragrances are preferable because they can produce the same aroma, and thus the same product, over and over again. It does not matter to the food industry that the therapeutic effects of a particular oil are no longer effective!

Other factors affecting the quality of oils

Like good wines, good oils have a vintage and a vineyard! Plants and essential oils, just like grapes and the wine they eventually produce, are affected by where, when and how they are grown. They are influenced by similar factors: the climate, the location where the plants are grown, the source of the plant, the quality of the cultivation process, when the plant is harvested and how it is looked after once it is harvested. In some cases this produces chemotypes.

What are chemotypes?

Chemotypes are botanically identical plants that produce chemically different oils. So two lavender plants may look exactly the same but the chemical composition of their oils will vary. This is caused by the factors mentioned above: where and when they are grown, the climate, soil quality, time of harvest and techniques used (e.g. by hand or machine) and the quality of the cultivation. If this difference in chemical make-up alters the oil's properties and effects, this is known as a chemotype and the oil may be labelled as such. It is worth remembering that chemotypes are not unnatural and have not been adulterated in any way: they are just chemically different because they have consistently been grown in a particular place or for a specific reason. So, for example, essential oil specialists may sell lavender plus a chemotype lavender, one may be grown at a high altitude and the other at sea level: the difference in altitude affects the chemical composition.

● Useful Tip

To try and remember what a chemotype is think about wine! Wine comes from grapevines and depending on where the vines are grown the grapes and the wine they produce will be completely different. An Australian white wine that uses the same grape variety, like chardonnay, as a French white wine will taste very different: in some senses they are chemotypes.

3 How aromatherapy works

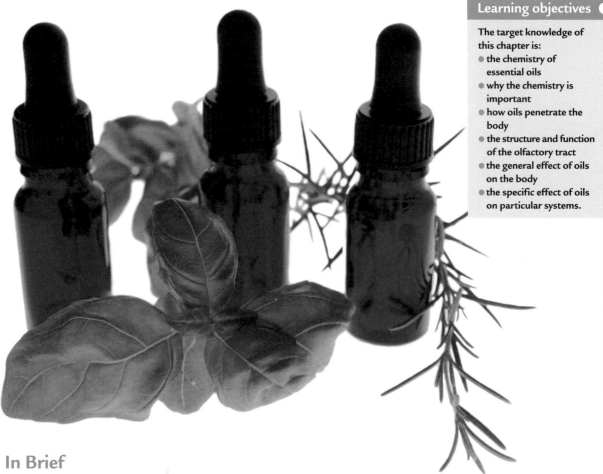

Learning objectives

The target knowledge of this chapter is:
- the chemistry of essential oils
- why the chemistry is important
- how oils penetrate the body
- the structure and function of the olfactory tract
- the general effect of oils on the body
- the specific effect of oils on particular systems.

In Brief

The name aromatherapy might make you think that this treatment works solely through the aromas, i.e. the smells, of plants. However, although the smell of a plant or herb is very important for the therapy to be effective (for example, if a patient doesn't like the smell of an oil the treatment is unlikely to work very well!) it is not the only factor to consider. Essential oils are very complex chemical structures and in order to understand their properties and effects (i.e. what they do and thus how to use them) it is helpful to know a little about their chemistry.

THE CHEMISTRY OF ESSENTIAL OILS

Humans have a very complicated chemical structure and so do the fluids that flow around their bodies. This is the same for plants: they are complicated chemical structures and so are their fluids, including essential oils which some people refer to as the 'life force'. The following section explains a little about the chemistry of these oils.

How does a plant grow?

When we think of the growth of a living structure, whether a plant or a human, we think of it getting bigger and developing. What enables this change in size or structure is chemicals. Everything around us, whether organic (living) or not (inorganic) is made of chemicals and growth happens because the chemical structure of a living thing is developing.

For example, humans and plants are made of three main chemical elements: carbon, hydrogen and oxygen plus thousands of trace elements. Humans take these chemicals into their body, by breathing (air), drinking (water) and eating, and make proteins with them which are used for growth and repair. Plants absorb the chemical elements found in soil, in water and in air (carbon, hydrogen, oxygen, nitrogen and other elements) and use these to make proteins, for growth and repair, carbohydrates and essential oils. The natural process of turning simple elements into complex chemical groups is known as *biosynthesis*.

So how does a plant make chemicals into leaves and flowers?

Every leaf and flower is made of millions of tiny fragments of chemical elements known as atoms. These atoms link up to make groups of atoms known as molecules which, in turn, join together to form all the different parts of a plant: its leaves, its flowers and its essential oil.

In plants, the link between a simple element – e.g. an atom of carbon or an atom of hydrogen on its own – and a complex group – e.g. a collection of atoms joined together, known as a *molecule* – is the energy of the sun. The sun's energy is captured by the plant's chlorophyll (the green pigment in the leaves) and used to convert the carbon dioxide in the air into other organic substances, in a process known as photosynthesis. Carbon and oxygen are the products of this: the carbon is used to make organic compounds (hydrocarbons and sugars) and some of the oxygen is released. The plant then uses this sugar to feed itself and grow. Plants also take the chemical elements in water and the soil, break them down into simple elements and then convert them into organic compounds it can use. This is called biosynthesis.

These basic metabolisms keep a plant alive. However, further metabolic changes occur in the plant, and one of the products of these is essential oil.

The symbols are used to represent atoms of carbon, hydrogen and oxygen.

C H O

What is an atom?

An atom is the smallest possible unit of a chemical element. It is microscopic and attaches itself to other atoms in order to make bigger structures, known as molecules.

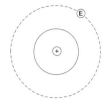

Ⓔ *electron*
⊕ *proton*

An atom of hydrogen

What is a molecule?

A molecule is a structure made of two or more atoms joined together. Molecules have particular qualities depending on how much of each chemical element they contain and the way in which those elements are arranged i.e. their shape. Each plant, and in particular each essential oil, has a different combination of molecules arranged in a different pattern. In a way a plant is a combination of different ingredients and it is this chemical 'recipe' and its arrangement which gives each essential oil its individual aroma, therapeutic qualities and effects.

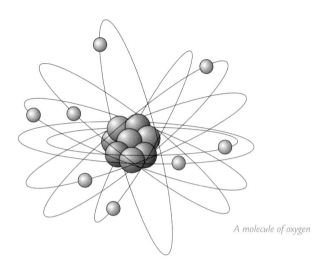

A molecule of oxygen

Why are molecules of any interest to the aromatherapist?

Each molecule of an essential oil produces a particular effect and has a specific therapeutic quality. Thus, if an aromatherapist knows which oil, or which family of oils, contain which molecules, she/he will understand which oils to use for particular treatments. The seven groups of molecules that are important to the aromatherapist, specifically because their effects and actions have been studied, are *terpenes, sesquiterpenes, esters, aldehydes, ketones, alcohols, phenols, oxides* and *acids*. Terpene molecules, which are made of the atoms of hydrogen and carbon joined together, are known as hydrocarbons whereas all the other molecule groups contain oxygen as well as hydrogen and carbon and are known as oxygenated compounds. The following list gives the main properties and effects of each group.

Terpenes
- found in most essential oils
- antiviral e.g. limonene (in citrus oils like grapefruit, lemon, mandarin)
- antiseptic e.g. pinene (in juniper and pine)
- anti-inflammatory, bactericidal e.g. chamazulene (in blue, or German, and Roman chamomile).

Esters
- fungicidal and relaxing e.g. linalyl acetate (in neroli and clary sage); geranyl acetate (in marjoram).

Aldehydes
- common in lemon-scented oils
- antiseptic e.g. citral (in bergamot and lemongrass)
- sedative.

Ketones
- often poisonous and several oils containing them, e.g. pennyroyal, are banned from use

Did you know?

Water is a molecule which links two atoms of hydrogen (H_2) with one atom of oxygen (O): its chemical make-up is thus H_2O. Of course, when you turn on a tap, it is not just one molecule coming out but millions!

Useful Tip

Remember these molecules with the mnemonic TEAKA-POSA – formed from the first letter of each name.

- decongestants, thus used for upper respiratory problems e.g. thujone (found in clary sage – generally used in preference to sage which is more toxic)
- safe ketones: jasmone (in jasmine) and fenchone (in fennel).

Alcohols

- antiseptic, antiviral, uplifting e.g. linalol (in bergamot, basil, ylang ylang); menthol (in peppermint); geraniol (in neroli, geranium, lavender).

Phenols

- bactericidal, stimulating e.g. thymol (in thyme), eugenol – (in clove and cinnamon)
- may irritate skin
- most, when isolated, are toxic so it is wise to be extra careful when using any essential oils containing them.

Oxides

- expectorant e.g. cineol (in eucalyptus, marjoram, rosemary).

Sesquiterpenes

- a form of terpene, with the same qualities and effects e.g. chamazulene (in Roman and blue chamomile).

Acids

- rarely found in essential oils and only in tiny amounts
- anti-inflammatory.

Do synthetic oils have the same effects?

No, because synthetics are rarely exact copies. Most oils are a mixture of two or three chemical elements plus many trace elements (i.e. tiny amounts of other elements). It is the synergy between the main components and the traces, i.e. how all the different molecules work together as a whole oil, which is important. Since exact components of oils are not known, it is impossible to make copies that work as effectively as the real thing.

You now know the basic chemistry of essential oils. This will help you to understand the effect of different oils and make connections between oils from the same plant family with similar molecular structures. The next section explains how aromatherapy works.

HOW ESSENTIAL OILS AND AROMATHERAPY WORK ON THE HUMAN BODY

In order to understand how essential oils work on the body, it is helpful to remember that we are complex chemical beings full of fluids, especially water. It is therefore logical that essential oils, which are also complex chemical fluids, are likely to affect our own body chemistry.

What are the specific effects of aromatherapy?

Using essential oils affects the human body –

- **pharmacologically**: essential oils are chemical and so are humans. Once

essential oils have been absorbed into the body, either through the skin or inhalation, the chemicals in the oils enter the blood and other body fluids and interact with the chemistry of our bodies. For example, hormones, enzymes and neurotransmitters (which enable the nervous system to work) are all chemicals and the presence of another chemical (the essential oil) can affect the way they work.

- **physiologically**: physiology is the way our body works. Essential oils can affect this by changing the chemical messages and impulses sent around the body and thus changing the way the systems of the human body function. For example, if an oil has relaxing and de-stressing properties, it may help to relieve the symptoms of stress displayed by our bodies e.g. slowing heart rate and breathing rate or encouraging tense muscles to relax.

- **psychologically**: the way essential oils affect our mind is more difficult to describe, mainly because everyone's mind is different. However, our sense of smell is closely linked to our memory so that particular smells can cause particular responses: for example, if you dislike the smell of roses, rose oil is unlikely to relax you; if jasmine reminds you of a good holiday then its smell will bring back happy memories and provoke a positive response.

The general effects of aromatherapy

There are certain general effects from using essential oils which result from most treatments, especially since relaxing and/or hands-on application methods like massage and baths are very common in aromatherapy. General effects include:

- reduction in stress and tension
- feeling of well-being, balance and calm
- antibacterial effects of oil help the body to heal and support the immune system.

How do essential oils penetrate the body?

There are two ways that oils can safely penetrate the body: smell/inhalation (through the nose) and absorption (through the skin). Ingestion (swallowing them) is not safe.

Smelling and inhaling essential oils: the nose and olfactory tract

Smell is the fastest way for essential oils to penetrate the body. The molecules travel up the nose and there are two results: they send a message to the brain and nerves which respond to the new smell and they pass into the bloodstream via the lungs and respiratory system. In order to understand how this works, it helps to understand the structure of the olfactory tract.

Structure

Most of the nose is concerned with breathing: inhaling air into the body and exhaling it from the body. However, it is also the organ of smell and thus very important in a therapy based on the power of aromas! At the top of the nose

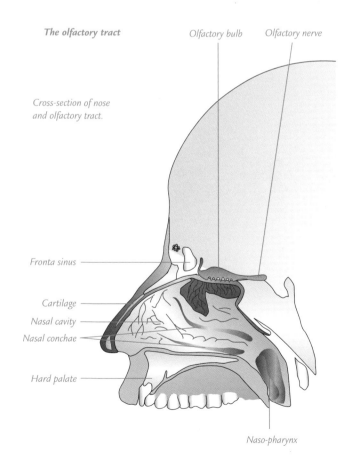

The olfactory tract   Olfactory bulb   Olfactory nerve

Cross-section of nose and olfactory tract.

Fronta sinus

Cartilage

Nasal cavity

Nasal conchae

Hard palate

Naso-pharynx

there are two areas of pigmented tissue known as olfactory membranes. They contain the olfactory, or smell-sensing cells, which have fine hair-like protrusions called cilia. The olfactory cells connect to nerves in an area known as the olfactory plexus. Once triggered, these nerves send messages along the olfactory nerves to the brain, particularly the limbic system. This area of the brain deals with memory, emotions, our basic instincts and mechanical functions.

Function

When the essential oil molecules pass over the olfactory cells, it is thought that these cells trigger receptor areas which send an impulse via the olfactory plexus and nerves to the brain. Here the information is processed and interpreted (i.e. is it a new smell, a nice smell, a smell with positive or negative associations?).

Depending on the interpretation, the brain sends messages to other parts of the body to elicit a response (e.g. if dislike is the message the person will stop sniffing the bottle, possibly grimace, and turn away from the smell). The brain may also react to different chemicals in an essential oil and produce particular effects: e.g. a relaxing or sedative substance may cause the brain to send out a message of relaxation either to the whole body or a particular part.

How do oils penetrate the skin?

Essential oils are absorbed through the skin. In order to understand this, it helps to understand the skin's structure. The skin is the largest human organ and it covers the body. It is water-resistant, but extremely minute substances, such as the molecules of an essential oil, can enter the tiny pores of the epidermis, the skin's surface layer, as well as penetrating through the hair follicles and the sweat glands. From the hair follicles and sweat glands, they enter the blood capillaries in the dermis, the skin's second layer. Once the oil reaches the blood and the circulation it is transported around the whole body.

Isn't it faster and thus more effective to swallow oils?

Essential oils should never be swallowed, even when diluted. There are several reasons for this. First, essential oils can be toxic. Second, they are extremely concentrated and, if swallowed, can damage the lining of the stomach. Third, the enzymes in the stomach change the chemical structure of the oils and thus change their therapeutic effect or prevent them from working. Fourth, they put a strain on the liver which works to remove them and fifth they become weaker as they pass through the digestive system. Finally, it is much slower, not faster, to absorb an oil through the digestive system rather than through the skin or

Cross-section of skin

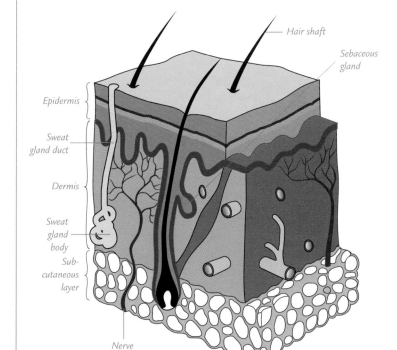

Hair shaft

Sebaceous gland

Epidermis

Sweat gland duct

Dermis

Sweat gland body

Sub-cutaneous layer

Nerve

inhalation (where, in both cases, it enters the bloodstream more directly). It is best to think of aromatherapy as an external treatment which has internal effects.

You now know how aromatherapy works and how it affects the body in general. The next section explains the specific benefits and effects of aromatherapy for particular systems of the body.

HOW DO ESSENTIAL OILS AFFECT THE BODY'S INDIVIDUAL SYSTEMS?

Though the effect of a particular oil is generally integral (i.e. applies to the whole body not just one part) it is possible to describe how each system is specifically affected by aromatherapy.

The skin

Aromatherapy massage treatments and baths affect the skin directly because massage involves rubbing oils into the skin and baths involve soaking the skin in water containing oils. So no matter what problem or part of the body is being treated, the skin will benefit, gaining:

- improved elasticity which helps to promote healing of scar tissue, reduce stretch marks; increased softness and suppleness
- faster desquamation (the flaking off of dead skin cells) which encourages the growth of new cells in the basal layer of the dermis as well as promoting a healthier, clearer skin tone.

Treatments for different skin types

Specific essential oil treatments for the skin depend on the problem being treated and/or the skin type. However, since many aromatherapy treatments involve massage of the skin, it is useful to know how to treat different skin types. The four main skin types are dry, sensitive, oily and dehydrated and each one benefits from particular oils. Before using any oils, a patch test is recommended: massage a small amount of the prepared essential oil (blended in either a carrier oil or cream) into the crook of the elbow or behind the ear.

Leave for 24 hours and check for reactions.

Dry

Dry skin suffers from a lack of sebum, a natural oil which is produced by the sebaceous glands in the dermis. It often wrinkles and loses elasticity faster than oily skin. Oils which stimulate the sebaceous glands help to increase the skin's natural lubrication and make the skin more healthy. Dry skin also tends to be sensitive and the oils used for sensitive skin (see below) are useful. For dry skin use:

- geranium
- lavender
- sandalwood
- rose
- jasmine
- chamomile

NB All references to chamomile, unless stated otherwise, will refer to blue, or German chamomile.

- carrot seed
- neroli.

Sensitive

Sensitive skin is extremely reactive to heat, cold, beauty products and, sometimes, massage. Before using any oils on sensitive skin, a patch test is recommended: if there are no abnormal reactions treatment is possible but only using very low concentrations of essential oils. The following oils are all very gentle and suitable for use:

- chamomile
- sandalwood
- neroli
- rose.

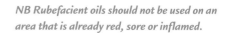

The aromatherapist should be especially careful when using absolutes of these oils, since the solvent used to extract them may cause skin irritation.

Oily

In direct contrast to dry skin, oily skin produces too much sebum and is over-lubricated. The most effective treatments use oils that help to control sebum production e.g.

- bergamot
- lavender
- lemon.

In severe cases, oily skin may develop acne. The following oils are beneficial for treating this condition:

- bergamot
- lavender
- geranium
- ylang ylang
- tea tree

NB Citrus oils may be phototoxic and this should be taken into account when using them to treat the skin.

Other oils which benefit the skin include:

- lemongrass
- rosemary.

The vascular system

No matter which method of applying essential oils is used, the oils will eventually find their way into the blood and be transported around the body. Certain oils have a particular effect on the blood and the circulation –

- Rubefacient oils – also known as 'warming' oils, these oils warm the tissues in the area of application. This allows the blood vessels in that area to dilate, enabling a more efficient circulation. Thus the delivery of oxygen and food and the removal of waste are faster which helps to speed up healing. Rubefacients include black pepper, rosemary, ginger, lemon and eucalyptus.

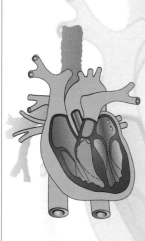

Cross-section of the heart.

NB Rubefacient oils should not be used on an area that is already red, sore or inflamed.

- Hypotensive oils – these oils lower blood pressure and are very efficient for treating high blood pressure (hypertension). They also have calming and relaxing effects, thus reducing blood pressure even further. Hypotensives oils include lavender, marjoram, ylang ylang and lemon.

- Hypertensive oils – low blood pressure is as dangerous as high blood pressure and hypertensive oils help to stimulate and invigorate the circulation, thus increasing pressure and aiding the prevention of other circulatory problems such as chilblains. Hypertensives include rosemary, black pepper, eucalyptus and ginger.

- Tonics – oils with a tonic, cooling effect have an opposite effect to that of rubefacient oils. They help to constrict capillaries thus reducing swellings and inflammations. Tonics include cypress, lemon and chamomile.

The skeletal and muscular systems

Joints and muscles benefit from oils with a rubefacient effect. The blood, warmed and stimulated by the oil, moves faster, bringing oxygen to stiff or immobile muscles and joints and thus helping to remove lactic acid build-ups and waste such as carbon dioxide. Detoxifying oils, such as juniper, lemon, fennel can help to reduce the uric acid build-up that causes gout as well as relieving the symptoms of other forms of arthritis, such as inflammation and swelling.

Lateral view of the skeleton

Helpful treatments include:

- rubefacients: black pepper, rosemary, ginger, lemon, eucalyptus. *NB None of these oils should be used on an area that is already red, sore or inflamed.*
- depurative (detoxifying): fennel, lemon, juniper.

The lymphatic system

The lymphatic system helps the circulation by collecting any excess tissue fluid that the blood capillaries can't carry, filtering it and returning it to the blood. It is especially important for the body's immunity because antibodies and bacteria-eating cells are produced in lymphatic tissue. Stimulating the lymphatic system thus stimulates two processes: the production of antibodies and the filtering of tissue fluid to remove waste and potentially harmful micro-organisms. Oils that stimulate the lymphatic system can be used preventatively, to strengthen the body's own defences or to treat particular conditions caused by an ineffective lymphatic system, like the build-up of cellulite, water retention and bloating. Useful oils include–

- lymphatic stimulants: geranium, juniper, rosemary
- eliminating oils (for cellulite, bloating): grapefruit, fennel, lemon, carrot seed
- diuretics (for fluid retention): chamomile, fennel, juniper.

The nervous system

The nervous system is the body's communication and instruction network. Think of it as a very complex wiring arrangement rather like a telephone system linking every area of the body. It is able to send and receive messages to every cell ensuring optimum functioning under all circumstances. It warns the body of danger and sends messages regarding pain and all sensations. Often the nervous system works to protect us by coordinating various body functions and physical and mental reactions. Sometimes a non-physical danger can occur which can produce the sensations of worry or stress. The body has a tendency to react to these sensations in the same way as if a physical danger had occurred, e.g. keeping the body in a state of heightened nervousness, anxious and full of adrenaline, ready to react if necessary. In the long term, this can cause tension, restlessness, an inability to relax and insomnia. In more serious cases, high blood pressure and heart problems may develop. Aromatherapy can relax an over-active nervous system and, where pain is felt, slow down the reactions of pain receptors and thus reduce the pain.
Useful oils include –

- analgesics: painkillers e.g. chamomile, lavender, rosemary, clary sage
- antispasmodics: calm nerves which tell muscles to go into spasms e.g. chamomile, ginger, marjoram
- sedatives: slow down activity thus help relieve insomnia, stress, tension e.g. lavender, chamomile, bergamot, ylang ylang
- stimulants: get systems going, for use in cases of convalescence and weakness e.g. basil (used with care), peppermint, ylang ylang
- nervines: help the whole nervous system e.g. rosemary, marjoram and melissa.

NB Some oils have a mixture of properties and can be used for several nervous conditions.

Centre: Cross-section of a lymphatic node.

A nerve cell.

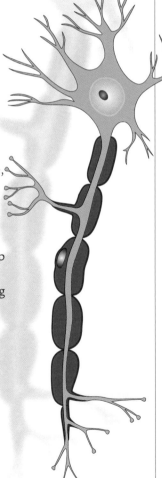

HOW AROMATHERAPY WORKS

The endocrine system

The endocrine system, like the nervous system, is a communication network. It uses chemicals in the forms of hormones to tell the body to grow, change and behave in certain ways. Aromatherapy can help this system in several different ways:

- may help control over/under-production of certain hormones, especially those from the thyroid gland and the adrenal cortex (e.g. basil, geranium and rosemary oils)
- balancing the hormones used in the reproductive system, thus relieving menopausal/menstrual problems (e.g. fennel – used with care, clary sage, cypress, chamomile, rose)
- may help control high, and thus potentially dangerous blood sugar levels (e.g. geranium, eucalyptus, juniper)
- may help control appetite (e.g. bergamot).

The reproductive system

Essential oils are very useful for treating the problems associated with pre-menstrual tension (depression, anxiety, fluid retention, cramps) and the menopause. However, pregnant women should avoid many essential oils because they are abortifacients (cause abortions) and emmenagogues (provoke menstruation). Helpful treatments include –

- geranium for pre-menstrual tension
- rose, geranium, jasmine for menopausal problems
- jasmine for prostate problems
- chamomile, fennel, juniper, geranium, cypress for fluid retention (PMT)
- rose for re-establishing balance.

NB Essential oils should never be used in the first three months of pregnancy. For the rest of the term, mandarin is the only oil that is recommended for use and only in weak dilution.

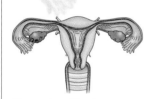

Cross-section of female reproductive system.

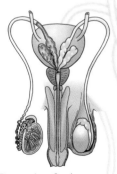

Cross-section of male reproductive system.

The digestive system

Essential oils should not be taken internally but they can be used externally to help the digestive system. Baths and massage of the abdomen both help intestinal problems such as diarrhoea, indigestion and constipation. Also, the inhalation of oils affects the digestive system indirectly because the molecules of essential oils are carried to it in the circulation. Useful oils include –

- antispasmodics (prevent pain and spasm): chamomile, clary sage, sweet fennel, peppermint, lavender
- stimulants: black pepper, orange, sweet fennel, ginger
- eliminating oils (especially for flatulence): chamomile, fennel, marjoram.

The respiratory system

One of the most effective ways of using essential oils is to inhale them, either from a tissue that has been impregnated with drops of oil, in a steam inhalation, from bath water or in the vapours from a burner or diffuser. The essential oil molecules cause impulses to be sent to the brain (see p. 23 'Smelling and inhaling essential oils: the nose and olfactory tract'). The brain can then send responses, which may affect various parts of the body. Using essential oils in this way will also allow some of the oil molecules to dissolve in the mucus that lines the respiratory tract. These will then be absorbed into the body's fluids and diffused throughout the body. Many oils have the ability to irritate mucus membranes and a good working knowledge of essential oils is necessary to avoid reactions. It is difficult to do a patch test up the nose!

The respira passages fro pharynx to bronchi.

No matter which method of aromatherapy treatment is used, smelling and breathing in the oils is an important factor. For example, during massage, oils penetrate the skin in a blend or a cream but the smell of the oils used will also have an effect. Thus the respiratory system, like the skin, can benefit directly or indirectly from aromatherapy treatments. Specific treatments to help respiratory problems like asthma, bronchitis, coughs, colds, flu and pneumonia include –

- antispasmodics: bergamot, chamomile, lavender
- decongestants: frankincense, eucalyptus
- antiseptics (for infections): bergamot, lavender, eucalyptus, tea tree
- expectorants (encourage coughing and clearing of mucus): bergamot, eucalyptus, lavender, sandalwood
- general cold remedies: eucalyptus, lavender, marjoram (white thyme for sore throats).

The urinary system

The urinary system is the body's liquid waste removal unit. It is often subject to bacterial infections – in the bladder (cystitis), kidneys and urinary tract and aromatherapy can be used to treat the symptoms and effects of these problems. Antiseptic oils can help to clear infections, diuretic oils can be used to encourage urine production and thus help wash away bacteria and certain oils are effective in relieving the symptoms of kidney infections, although medical advice should be sought before treating any kidney problem. Useful oils include –

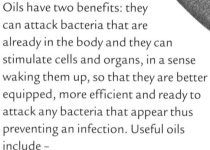

- antiseptics: bergamot, chamomile, eucalyptus, tea tree
- diuretics: cypress, fennel, juniper, chamomile.

Above: Cross-section of a kidney.

The immune system

An immune system that is working properly can help to stop the body becoming ill in the first place. Due to their antiseptic and antiviral qualities, regular use of essential oils can help to strengthen the body's immunity and prevent infection and disease. Most oils have some antibacterial qualities. Oils have two benefits: they can attack bacteria that are already in the body and they can stimulate cells and organs, in a sense waking them up, so that they are better equipped, more efficient and ready to attack any bacteria that appear thus preventing an infection. Useful oils include –

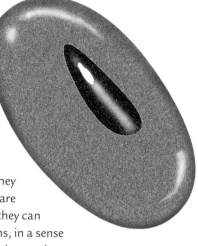

A cell.

- antibacterial: bergamot, eucalyptus, rosemary, tea tree, lavender
- febrifuges (reduce fever): eucalyptus, peppermint, tea tree
- sudorifics (promote sweating): rosemary, white thyme
- overall immune system stimulants: lavender, bergamot, tea tree
- lymphatic system stimulants: rosemary, geranium.

You now know all the aspects of aromatherapy function: the chemistry of essential oils and why this is important for oils to work effectively; how oils penetrate the body; the general effects of oils on the whole body and the effect of oils on specific systems.

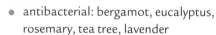

4 Application: buying and using oils

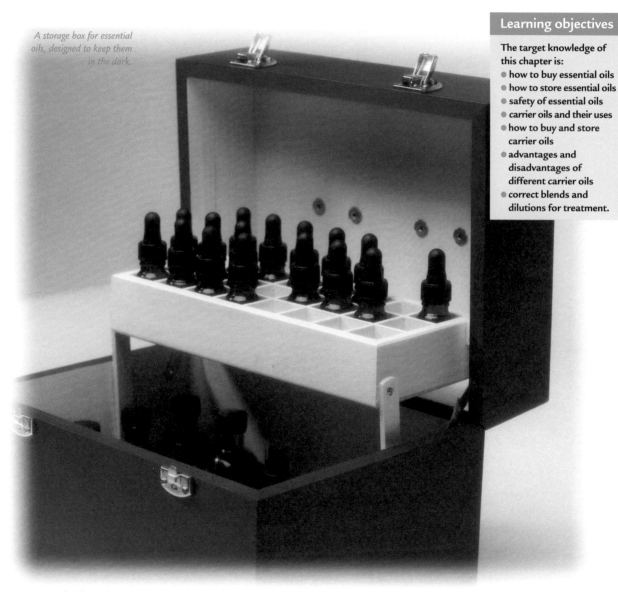

A storage box for essential oils, designed to keep them in the dark.

In Brief

This chapter provides information on buying and storing essential and carrier oils, the advantages and disadvantages of using different carrier oils, blending oils for massage and treatments and recommended dilutions.

BUYING AND STORING OILS

Before explaining how to use essential oils it is important to explain how not to use them! The first consideration for anyone planning to use essential oils is where to buy them.

How and where do I buy essential oils?

The most important factor to consider when buying essential oils is who supplies them. With a good, reliable supplier, there is no need to worry about the purity, origin or quality of the oils. The checklist below will help in selecting a supplier: a reputable source will be able to provide all the required information.

- Where is the oil from? What country and which region of that country?
- Was the plant organically grown?
- Which part of the plant was used to produce the oil?
- What is the plant's botanical name (usually in Latin)?
- How was the essential oil extracted: distillation, solvent extraction or expression?

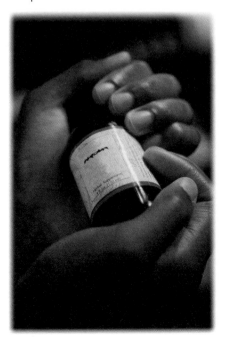

- How long has the oil been in stock?
- Where are the oils stored/are the oils stored properly? (if you are in the shop/warehouse you can check this) i.e. away from extremes of temperature.

Also, be aware of the following –

- are the oils unusually cheap? If so, they might not be the real thing. For example, if rose or jasmine oils are not much more expensive than rosemary or thyme, they might be blends or dilutions...rose and jasmine are extremely expensive.
- buy the best you can afford. The better the quality the better the effect.
- check that the oils are not synthetics, adulterations or 'nature-identical' copies: the positive effects of an essential oil cannot be exactly synthesised and aromatherapy treatments using artificial or diluted oils will be just as artificial, ineffective and weak!

How should oils be stored?

Essential oils are delicate and expensive. It is therefore wise to look after them. They should be stored –

- away from extremes of temperature: heat will evaporate them and cold can affect their composition
- in dark, amber glass bottles (or dark blue glass bottles if kept in the dark or a fridge): essential oils are sensitive to ultraviolet light; they should not be stored, or bought, in plastic because it affects the molecular structure of the oil
- in tightly sealed bottles: to protect them from evaporating in the air and to stop contact with the air from changing their composition
- out of the reach of children (childproof caps are now available for use with essential oil bottles).

THE SAFETY OF ESSENTIAL OILS

Are essential oils safe?
Used correctly, essential oils are very safe, mainly because they are used in such tiny amounts. When used in the wrong dilutions and in the wrong conditions they can produce adverse effects. Certain oils should never be used under any circumstances (see list below) and some should not be used for specific conditions.

NB Essential oils are very strong and should not be swallowed. If oil gets into an eye rinse it immediately with lots of water. If necessary seek medical advice.

When should oils not be used?
The effects of certain oils can be positive for some conditions and not for others. Problems can be avoided in three ways:
- consulting with clients to find out as much about their medical history and any contraindications
- knowing the properties and effects of all oils used
- using the oils in their correct and safe dilutions.

Specific conditions
Pregnancy
Avoid oils which have the following properties –
- emmenagogues: provoke menstruation
- diuretics: provoke urine production
- parturients: provoke parturition i.e. childbirth
- abortifacient: cause abortions
- uterine stimulants: cause the uterus to constrict thus provoking abortions.

NB Essential oils should never be used in the first three months of pregnancy. For the rest of the term, mandarin is the only oil which should be used.

Epilepsy
Never use
- sweet fennel
- rosemary.

General skin irritants
The following oils can irritate the skin so are not recommended for those with sensitive skin or anyone prone to skin allergies. It is also useful to remember that solvent-extracted oils will contain traces of the solvent used and may cause irritations.

Basil	*Melissa*
Black pepper	*Orange*
Clove	*Peppermint*
Ginger	*Thyme*
Lemon	*Tea tree*
Lemongrass	

Photosensitisation
Certain oils make the skin more sensitive to ultraviolet light and should be avoided before exposure to sunlight or before going on a sunbed –
- bergamot
- grapefruit (particularly if distilled)
- lemon
- mandarin
- patchouli
- lime (particularly if expressed)
- sweet orange.

Allergies
For anyone who is allergic or suspects an allergy to a particular oil, a skin test is recommended. Rub one drop of diluted oil into the crook of the arm or behind the ear and leave for 24 hours. If there is no reaction, the oil is probably safe to use once diluted as necessary.

Which oils should never be used?
Here is a list of toxic oils which should never be used, under any circumstances.

Aniseed	*Cinnamon bark*
Arnica	*Dwarf pine*
Bitter almond	*Elecampane*
Bitter fennel	*Horseradish*
Camphor	*Hyssop*
Cassia	*Mustard*

Origanum
Pennyroyal
Rue
Sage
Sassafras
Savin
Savory (winter and summer)

Southernwood
Tansy
Thuja
Wintergreen
Wormseed
Wormwood

You now know how to buy and store oils and which ones not to buy. The following section explains how to blend them for use.

BLENDING AND CARRIER OILS

Essential oils are almost always used in a blend. They are blended with carrier oils for use in massage and, in some cases, baths. The correct blend is very important because essential oils are potentially toxic if used undiluted. They are also highly concentrated and will therefore not go very far in a massage on their own!

What is a carrier oil?

Carrier oils are also known as fixed oils because, unlike essential oils, they do not evaporate when heated. They are extracted from plants, flowers, nuts and seeds. Those generally recommended for use in aromatherapy do not have a strong smell as it might interfere with that of the essential oil. Some carriers contain fat-soluble vitamins (e.g. A, D, E and K), minerals and proteins in different amounts depending on the oil, so some carrier oils have health benefits of their own. Carrier oils used in aromatherapy are –

- of vegetable, nut or seed origin
- refined, preferably cold-pressed, quality i.e. they have been extracted without the use of excessive heat which means they are purer and they retain their vitamin content
- stable, not volatile; unlike essential oils they do not evaporate on exposure to heat and light
- used neat

- non-sticky: heat and pressure (massage uses/produces both) can cause some oils to become sticky e.g. avocado; suitable carrier oils are smooth
- lubricants for aromatherapists' hands, giving a smooth massage.

Which oils are recommended?

There are several suitable carrier oils which can be used alone or in a blend with other carriers. Some are lighter than others and often the thicker, denser oils, which are more expensive, are used diluted with a lighter oil to make them go further. Lighter oils are better for full body massage because they allow smoother movements whereas the thicker oils are more useful for massage on a small area.

Recommended carrier oils:

Grapeseed
Sweet Almond
Wheatgerm
Evening primrose
Avocado (although does have a strong smell)
Jojoba (actually a liquid wax)
Calendula (actually an infused oil)
Macadamia
Peach kernel

Grapeseed (vitis vinifera)
From the seeds of grapes.

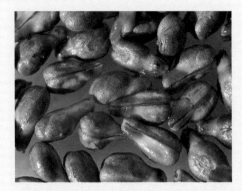

Properties
- finely-textured i.e. smooth, not grainy or sticky, flows freely
- high in linoleic acid (a poly-unsaturated fatty acid, essential to the body and good for helping prevent heart disease)
- contains some vitamin E (which helps the oil keep for longer and protects/nourishes the skin).

Advantages
- smooth: good for full body massage.

Disadvantages
- produced by hot extraction (the raw material is heated beyond 70 degrees to extract the oil), therefore it is not as pure as some other oils.

Sweet almond (prunus amygdalis var. dulcis)

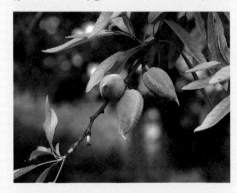

From the sweet almond nut (not to be confused with bitter almond which is toxic).

Properties
- contains high percentage of vitamins (A, B1, B2, B6) and mono- and polyunsaturated fatty acids (essential for the body to function)
- pale yellow in colour.

Advantages
- keeps well due to vitamin E content
- cold-pressed therefore relatively pure
- benefits skin: has protective and nourishing qualities.

Wheatgerm (triticum vulgare)
From the vitamin-rich 'germ' (i.e. the seed of the seed which will grow into wheat) of the wheat kernel.

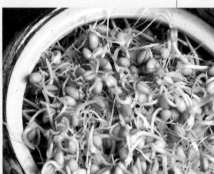

Properties
- stabilises other oils and blends because it is a natural antioxidant (oxidation is a chemical reaction caused by the presence of oxygen: for example rust is the result of a metal reacting with oxygen and moisture – an antioxidant slows or prevents the reaction and in the case of oils helps to preserve them); adding 5-10% wheatgerm oil to another carrier or a blend will help preserve it for a couple of months
- contains vitamin E
- orangey-brown in colour.

Advantages
- good for reducing scarring after operations
- useful on dry/mature skins.

Disadvantages
- too thick and sticky to use alone for massage: needs to be mixed with a light oil
- may cause allergies.

Evening primrose (oenothera biennis)

From evening primrose flower seeds.

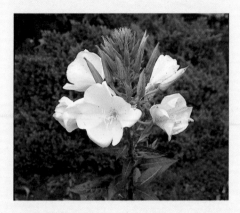

Properties

- contains linoleic acid and GLA (gammo-linoleic acid) which are both essential for the body but not made by it so must be provided by diet; GLA is also known to reduce the symptoms of pre-menstrual tension.

Advantages

- useful for treating dry skin conditions including eczema and dandruff
- useful for PMT.

Disadvantages

- expensive.

Avocado (persea americana)

From avocado fruits.

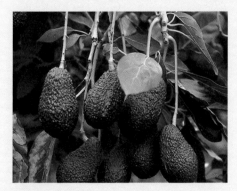

Properties

- contains lecithin (which contains phospholipids, which are an important part of all body membranes), saturated and monounsaturated fatty acids (essential for the body to function)
- high vitamin content: A, B, D
- dark green.

Advantages

- stores well (because it contains a natural antioxidant)
- emollient (softens and smooths skin)
- good for dry and/or wrinkled skin
- unrefined (which is why, when chilled, the oil sometimes turns cloudy)
- viscous but still penetrates the skin.

Disadvantages

- can become sticky during massage
- has a strong and distinctive smell.

Jojoba bean (simmondsia chinensis)

Jojoba is actually a liquid wax not a carrier oil. It can be a useful addition to a massage oil blend but is too expensive to be used as a base oil.

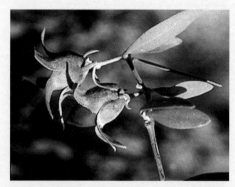

Properties

- fine-textured (smooth, not sticky or grainy)
- useful for many conditions: its chemical structure is similar to that of the skin's own oil, sebum, so it is useful for treating both excessive sebum production (oily skin and/or acne) because it can dissolve the sebum, as

well as underproduction, such as dry skin, dandruff or other dry skin conditions like eczema and psoriasis
- nourishing.

Advantages
- stable (i.e. does not evaporate or react easily with the air) so keeps well.

Disadvantages
- expensive.

Calendula (calendula officinalis)
Calendula is an infused oil and very different from a pure carrier oil. It has some useful properties in its own right but is used more in herbalism than aromatherapy.

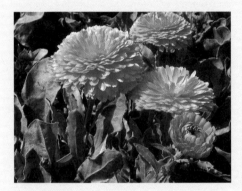

Properties
- anti-inflammatory
- anti-spasmodic
- healing.

Advantages
- healing qualities make it very suitable for skin problems (chapped skin, eczema, bruises, rashes) and sunburn.

Disadvantages
- not as pure as cold-pressed oils because of the maceration process.

Macadamia (macadamia integrifolia/ macadamia ternifolia)
From the macadamia nut.

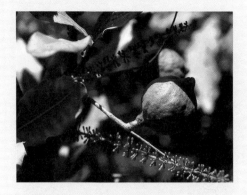

Properties
- good for dry/wrinkled skin (considered to be anti-ageing)
- emollient
- contains palmitoleic acid, also found in sebum (so therefore useful for treating both dry and oily skins)
- golden colour.

Advantages
- stable
- fine texture.

Peach kernel (prunus persica)
From the stone/seed of peaches.

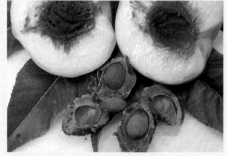

Properties
- similar (in terms of chemical structure and effects) to sweet almond and apricot kernel oils
- rich in vitamins (A, B1, B2, B6).

Advantages
- keeps well
- protects and nourishes skin.

Disadvantages
- expensive.

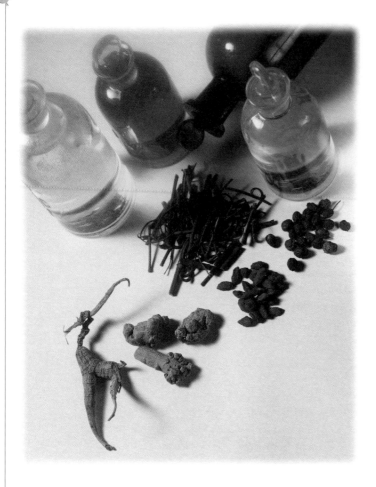

same care as essential oils. Do not make the mistake of using unsuitable oils like cooking oil (think of the aroma and consistency of most cooking oils when used: sticky, greasy and smelly!) or baby oil (this is a mineral oil, not a natural plant oil). Buy from a reputable supplier and, if possible, use oils which are organic and dated (i.e. when they were bottled because shelf lives vary).

How should they be stored?

Remember to –

- replace the bottle lids after use
- store in a cool place: they will go rancid in the heat just like butter left in the sun
- use the oldest first. Carrier oils have a limited shelf life (which varies according to the oil) so they need to be used before they go rancid.

What are the correct dilutions?

Dilutions depend on two factors: the treatment and the 'scale' of the treatment (i.e. is it for a full body massage, or just one part such as the face or feet?). The following are guidelines. The more experienced aromatherapist will adapt them according to circumstance and condition. Treat dilutions and blends like a medical treatment: a prescription must provide the right drug and dosage for the condition and patient. The same care should be used to create blends: use the right oils for the problem in the appropriate amounts. For a treatment to work, just like a prescription, the quantities and qualities of both essential and carrier oils must remain consistent.

How much essential oil should be mixed with a carrier oil?

Usually from 1% (weaker blend) to 2% (stronger blend). The maximum dilution should be 2.5% of essential oil.

Why use a carrier oil?

Carrier oils are the medium that, literally, carry the essential oil all over the body in a massage. It would be impossible to use essential oils undiluted for massage: they are not only dangerous (because they are so strong) and far too expensive but also ineffective because they are volatile and evaporate with the heat of the massage and in air/light. Carrier oils can slow down the evaporation rate of essential oils and help to transport the essential oil molecules all over the body to be gradually absorbed through the skin. Carrier oils themselves are only absorbed into the surface layers of the skin, because their molecules are too big to penetrate any deeper.

Where should I buy them?

Carrier oils should be bought with the

How do I work out and measure these percentages?

1% equals one drop essential oil to 100 drops carrier and 2% blend equals two drops essential oil to 100 drops carrier.

Do I have to count out 100 drops of a carrier oil?!

No. 100 drops of oil is equivalent to 5mls or one teaspoon. So 1% would be one drop of essential oil per teaspoon/5mls and 2% would be two drops of essential oil per teaspoon/5mls.

How much oil is needed for different treatments?

- Full body massages require about 20-25ml carrier oils. Dilute eight drops essential oil per 20mls carrier.
- For face massage, only about 5mls of carrier oil is needed. Dilute 1-2 drops essential oil per 5ml.
- Absolutes may contain traces of the solvents used in extracting them and thus a weaker dilution such as a 1% blend (i.e. one drop of an absolute to 100 drops/5ml) of carrier oil should be used.
- Baths: essential oils float or sink in water and are not diluted so drops should not be added directly to the water. Oils should be mixed with a small quantity of an emulsifier, such as a fragrance-free shampoo, bath gel, liquid soap or even full cream milk before adding to the bath. No more than six drops should be used per bath. Those with sensitive skin should use a lower concentration and special care should be taken with those essential oils known to cause skin irritations.
- Burners: use two drops of the chosen essential oil in water.
- Compresses: soak cloth in 100ml of water and add one drop of the chosen essential oil.
- Steam inhalations: use one drop of

essential oil to a bowl of hot water, or one or two more for a stronger effect. *(See Chapter 6 for more detailed information on using oils at home.)*

NB When using essential oils, always be careful not to overdose. If in doubt, don't.

Are there any instances when these dilutions are wrong or need changing?

Use a maximum 1% dilution when treating –
- clients with sensitive skin
- the elderly
- children
- the weak/convalescent
- pregnant or breastfeeding women.

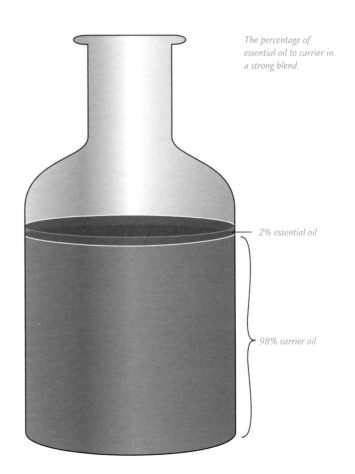

The percentage of essential oil to carrier in a strong blend.

2% essential oil

98% carrier oil

In general, blends should be adapted according to the strength of the smell of the essential oils used as well as the age and condition of the client. The amount of oil that needs to be blended is obviously dictated by the physical size of the client and which areas are being massaged. Someone with a larger frame will have more skin to massage! However, the dilution of the blend should never exceed 2.5%.

How long will the blend last?

The average shelf life of a blended oil, provided that the carrier oil is fresh, is approximately three months. If 10% of wheatgerm oil, a natural antioxidant, is added to the blend the shelf life should be six months. However, it is best to blend just enough oil for each individual treatment to avoid expense and waste.

Can oils be used undiluted?

Only in very specific circumstances, usually for antiseptic purposes i.e. using a few drops of neat lavender oil on a burn (like Gattefossé, the creator of aromatherapy, did), or dabbing tea tree oil onto a spot or skin blemish. A few drops of particular oils, especially those used for emotional effects like relaxation, stimulation or balance, can be placed onto a tissue and carried around for inhaling when necessary.

What is the maximum number of oils per treatment?

For the treatment of any one person a maximum of three essential oils should be used: two for the body and one for the face when required. Obviously, oils will mix in the body but certain oils are specifically recommended for treating skin types. No treatment should use more than eight drops of essential oil.

Does the treatment start working immediately?

The smell of an oil during any treatment will register in the brain and provoke a response within seconds. In massage, essential oils are primarily absorbed through the skin, and then into the body fluids. An area of skin is only able to absorb oils for about ten minutes after which it becomes saturated. The time taken for the oils to pass around the body is dictated by the individual metabolic rate and this varies from about twenty minutes to twelve hours. Most essential oils are processed and eliminated from the body within 24 hours although there are a few exceptions e.g. juniper and myrrh which both remain in the body for longer and therefore require careful use.

5 A-Z of essential oils

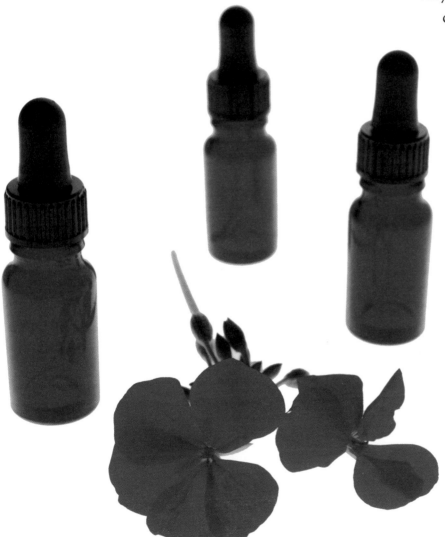

In Brief

The next chapter provides an easy reference guide to 42 of the most important essential oils.

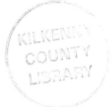

Learning objectives

The target knowledge of this chapter is:
- the therapeutic actions of essential oils
- the origins, properties and therapeutic uses of individual essential oils.

A–Z OF ESSENTIAL OILS

● A–Z EXPLAINED

Now that you have learnt what essential oils are and how to use them, you need to learn about the properties and effects of each individual oil. The oils are listed in alphabetical order.

Each listing includes the following –
● **botanical name** (useful for double-checking that what is contained in a bottle of oil is the real thing, not a substitute).

● **where** the plant comes from.

● which **part of the plant** is used for the oil (some plants produce several oils).

● **method of extraction**: useful because methods like solvent extraction leave a residue which can irritate the skin.

● **chemical make-up**: when you first encounter essential oils, their chemical make-up can be very confusing and difficult to understand. It may even seem irrelevant. However, gradually patterns begin to emerge and the different chemical constituents become recognisable. In a way it's a bit like a recipe: if something contains yeast it will rise, if it contains chilli it will be spicy, if it contains lots of sugar it will be sweet and if it contains lots of salt it will be salty. The same applies to the 'ingredients' of essential oils. So if you know that an oil contains a high proportion of terpenes, which are antiviral, stimulating and antiseptic, then you will know

that the oil has these qualities. Or if an oil contains a high proportion of alcohols, which are antiseptic and uplifting, the oil itself will be antiseptic and uplifting. Also, once you know that one plant from a particular group contains terpenes, alcohols or esters, and has the qualities connected with those chemicals, it is likely that another plant from that group will have a similar chemical make-up and effects. For example, most citrus oils contain a high proportion of a terpene called limonene. Terpenes are antiviral, antiseptic and invigorate the body so all citrus oils will have strong antiseptic and invigorating qualities. Indeed, any oil containing limonene will have those effects to a greater or lesser extent depending on the proportion it contains. In each entry the main chemicals contained are listed and a simple formula, using the letters of the molecules (T for terpenes, E for esters, AC for alcohols, K for ketones, AL for aldehydes, P for phenols, O for oxides, S for sesquiterpenes, A for acids) is provided to help the user learn each oil's contents.

● **therapeutic actions**: the effects of the oil on the body. You will notice that some oils are listed with apparently contradictory actions (for example stimulating and relaxing). This is because they have such complex chemical compositions that one molecule may act in one way on the body whereas another may cause a

completely opposite reaction. However, this does not mean that a treatment used for relaxation will be cancelled out by itself. An oil's molecules will be stimulated by the oils it is mixed with and how it is applied/used: these will determine the final outcome of the treatment.

● **conditions and systems that benefit from using the oil**: these list conditions that the oil has been shown to help but they are not meant to be exclusive. Experimenting (taking into account any safety factors or contraindications) with oils and blends is the best way to find out what works best for each individual.

● **safety factors**: contraindications to an oil's use are listed here. It should be noted that very few oils are recommended for use during pregnancy and that epileptics and those with blood pressure problems should take extra care.

● **if you remember only one thing...**: though it is impossible to sum up the benefits of any one oil, this last section gives a thumbnail description of its positive qualities.

GLOSSARY OF THERAPEUTIC ACTIONS

- **Analgesic**: painkilling effect
- **Anti-acid**: reduces the effects caused by too much gastric acid
- **Anti-allergic**: prevents allergic reactions
- **Anticatarrhal**: helps remove catarrh
- **Antidepressant**: helps lift depression and symptoms related to it
- **Anti-inflammatory**: reduces inflammations
- **Antimicrobial**: an agent which resists or destroys pathogenic micro-organisms
- **Antipruritic**: relieves sensation of itching or prevents its occurrence
- **Antiseptic**: prevents or removes infection
- **Antispasmodic**: calms, slows muscle spasm
- **Antiviral**: kills virus, or helps prevent a virus developing
- **Aphrodisiac**: heightens sexual desire
- **Astringent**: contracts and tightens tissues, especially skin
- **Bactericidal**: kills bacteria
- **Balancing**: creates balance in emotions or in activity of part of the body
- **Calming**: has an overall calming effect
- **Carminative**: helps prevent flatulence
- **Cephalic**: clears and focuses the mind
- **Cicatrisant**: helps wounds heal
- **Cooling**: cools the area of application; reduces temperature
- **Cordial**: a stimulant and tonic
- **Cytophylactic**: cell-regenerator
- **Deodorant**: removes or masks unpleasant smells
- **Depurative**: removes impurities and toxins
- **Diuretic**: increases urine production
- **Emmenagogue**: provokes menstruation – useful for clients suffering from amenorrhoea (absence of periods) but contraindicated for pregnant women
- **Expectorant**: helps fluidify, thus remove, mucus from lungs and respiratory passages
- **Febrifuge**: reduces fever
- **Fungicidal**: destroys fungi
- **Galactagogue**: increases the secretion of breast milk
- **Haemostatic**: stops bleeding
- **Hypertensive**: increases blood pressure
- **Hypotensive**: lowers blood pressure
- **Immuno-stimulant**: stimulates the immune system
- **Laxative**: promotes evacuation of the bowel
- **Nervine**: strengthening and toning to the nerves and nervous system
- **Oestrogenic**: helps promote production of oestrogen
- **Prophylactic**: preventive of disease or infection
- **Relaxing**: has a general relaxing effect
- **Refreshing**: has a refreshing effect
- **Rubefacient**: warms and reddens the area of application, and subsequently the blood vessels in that area dilate
- **Sedative**: calms the nervous system
- **Stimulant**: stimulates a particular system or the whole body
- **Stomachic**: aids digestion, eases indigestion
- **Sudorific**: increases perspiration
- **Tonic**: invigorates and gives strength to a specific area or the whole body depending on the oil
- **Uplifting**: helps positive thinking, 'lifts' the emotions
- **Vasoconstrictive**: reduces dilation of capillaries (thus reducing blood flow to an area and the redness it causes)
- **Vasodilatory**: increases dilation of capillaries (thus warming and increasing the blood flow to an area causing it to redden)
- **Vermifuge**: expels intestinal worms
- **Vulnerary**: An agent which helps heal wounds and sores by external application
- **Warming**: produces feeling of warmth.

Basil

One of the best herbs for cooking, basil is also a versatile essential oil.

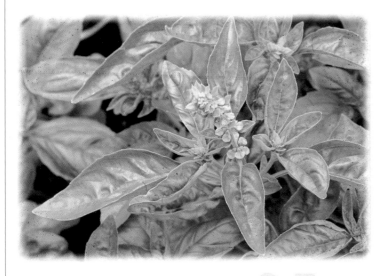

What is its botanical name?
Ocimum basilicum.

Where in the world does it come from?
Basil originates in Asia and Africa but is now found throughout the Mediterranean area of Europe (Italy and France) and in the USA.

Which part of the plant is used to make the oil?
The flowers and leaves of the herb.

How is it extracted?
By steam distillation.

What is its chemical make-up?
Basil is 40-45% linalol (Al-Cohol) and 23% methyl chavicol (P-henol). It also contains traces of eugenol (P-henol), limonene (T-erpene) and citronellol (Al-Cohol). Its chemical make-up is thus AC-P-T.

NB Methyl chavicol-free oil should be used where possible.

What are its general therapeutic actions?
Basil has the following actions:

- antiseptic
- antispasmodic
- cephalic
- emmenagogue
- tonic
- uplifting
- warming
- prophylactic.

Which conditions/systems benefit from using basil oil?

- *skin*: tonic effect on acne; reduces inflammation of wasp stings
- *muscular/digestive*: antispasmodic; relieves muscle tightness, especially in the intestines and stomach
- *nervous*: uplifting for depression, insomnia, stress; helps to focus the mind and aids concentration; headaches, migraine, fainting fits, neuralgia, neuritis
- *reproductive*: amenorrhoea (absence of periods) or irregular/scanty menstruation
- *respiratory*: sinusitis.

When shouldn't it be used?
On sensitive skins and pregnant women.

If you remember only one thing...
Basil is excellent for clearing the mind of worries and clutter and lifting one's spirit.

Benzoin

What is its botanical name?
Styrax benzoin.

Where in the world does it come from?
Sumatra, Java and Thailand.

Which part of the plant is used to make the oil?
The resin of the benzoin tree.

How is it extracted?
By solvent extraction and steam distillation.

What is its chemical make-up?
Benzoin is mostly coniferyl cinnamate (E-ster) and sumaresinolic acid (A-cid) combined with benzoic acid (A-cid) and traces of cinnamic acid (A-cid), vanillin (Al-Dehyde) and benzaldehyde (Al-Dehyde). Its chemical make-up is thus E-A-AD.

What are its therapeutic actions?
Benzoin has the following actions:
- carminative
- expectorant
- sedative
- cordial
- vulnerary
- warming.

Which conditions/systems benefit from its use?
- *skin*: reduces inflammations and relieves symptoms of dermatitis, cracked and chapped skin
- *skeletal*: warming effect reduces inflammation caused by rheumatoid arthritis and gout
- *circulatory*: warms heart and circulation and thus improves their efficiency
- *nervous*: stress, relieves tension
- *digestive*: aids digestion and relieves flatulence
- *urinary*: cystitis.

When shouldn't it be used?
Benzoin is relatively safe for use, though sensitive skins may react to it.

If you remember only one thing...
Benzoin creates a feeling of euphoria, and has a warming effect on the whole body, especially the heart, lungs and circulation.

Did you know?
Benzoin oil was once used in a product called Friar's Balsam, an inhalation used to ease respiratory problems.

Bergamot

What is its botanical name?
Citrus bergamia.

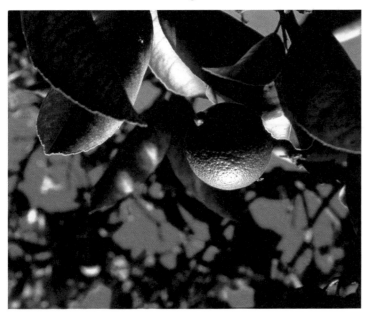

Where in the world does it come from?
It is native to tropical Asia but now cultivated in northern and southern Italy.

Which part of the plant is used to make the oil?
The rind/peel of the bergamot fruit, which resembles a miniature orange.

How is it extracted?
By expression.

What is its chemical make-up?
Bergamot is mainly 30-60% linalyl acetate (E-ster), 11-22% linalol (Al-Cohol) with traces of S-esquiterpenes and T-erpenes. Its chemical make-up is thus E-AC-S-T.

What are its therapeutic actions?
Bergamot has the following actions:
- analgesic
- anti-inflammatory
- antiseptic
- antiviral
- cooling
- relaxing
- sedative
- laxative
- vermifuge
- uplifting.

Which conditions/systems benefit from its use?
- *skin*: antiseptic, anti-inflammatory and cooling thus useful for treating many inflamed, sore skin conditions such as eczema, psoriasis and acne
- *nervous* (emotional): uplifting thus reduces anger, frustration, anxiety, stress and the symptoms of depression
- *digestive*: relieves flatulence, colic and painful digestion; helps regulate appetite
- *respiratory*: relieves symptoms of colds, flu and bronchitis as well as reducing inflammations and infections such as tonsillitis and sore throats
- *urinary*: cystitis
- *immune*: strengthens system.

When shouldn't it be used?
Before going into the sun or onto a sunbed since it increases sensitivity to ultraviolet light.
NB: Bergapten-free bergamot should be used where possible because bergapten is a furocoumarin which is the phototoxic ingredient. If the oil purchased is bergapten-free it will not be phototoxic but it will have been adulterated to remove the bergapten.

If you remember only one thing...
Like other citrus oils bergamot is uplifting and cheerful.

Black pepper

The black pepper we use on our food isn't quite the same as the essential oil; however, the oil does have the same spicy quality and can therefore be a skin irritant.

What is its botanical name?
Piper nigrum.

Where in the world does it come from?
India, Indonesia, Greece.

Which part of the plant is used to make the oil?
The dried berries.

How is it extracted?
By steam distillation.

What is its chemical make-up?
Black pepper is 70-80% T-erpenes (such as pinene, camphene, limonene and thujene) and 20-30% S-esquiterpenes. Its chemical make-up is T-S.

What are its therapeutic actions?
Black pepper is
- analgesic
- antispasmodic
- depurative
- expectorant
- rubefacient

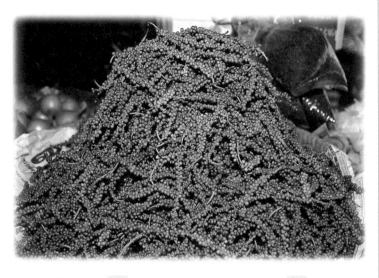

- stimulant
- tonic.

Which conditions/systems benefit from its use?
- *muscular*: tonic for aches and pains; can improve performance if used before sporting activities
- *circulatory/lymphatic*: warming thus stimulates circulation (thus preventing and relieving chilblains) and lymphatic system
- *nervous*: stimulates and thus strengthens the nerves and mind
- *digestive*: stimulates digestion and appetite; relieves bowel problems and constipation by aiding peristalsis
- *respiratory*: expectorant so relieves catarrh, coughs and colds.

When shouldn't it be used?
Black pepper can be irritating and should not be used neat on the skin. It is also incompatible with homeopathic treatments.

If you remember only one thing...
Black pepper warms the blood, thus relieving aches and pains in the muscles and stimulating the appetite.

Carrot seed

What is its botanical name?
Daucus carota.

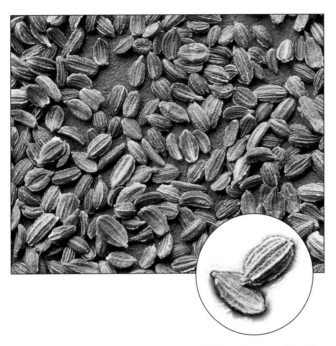

Where in the world does it come from?
Europe, Asia, North Africa.

Which part of the plant is used to make the oil?
Dried seeds.

How is it extracted?
Steam distillation.

What is its chemical make-up?
Carrot seed is mainly carotol, daucol, (both Al-Cohols), limonene and pinene (both T-erpenes). Its chemical make-up is thus AC-T.

What are its therapeutic actions?
Carrot seed is
- antiseptic
- depurative
- diuretic
- emmenagogue
- tonic
- vasodilatory.

Which conditions/systems benefit from its use?
- *skin*: tones and rejuvenates, good for mature, wrinkled skins and overheated, dry conditions and rashes, eczema, psoriasis, dermatitis
- *skeletal*: diuretic effect on build-up of uric acid that causes gout, rheumatism, arthritis
- *muscular*: detoxifies build-up of toxins in muscles
- *reproductive*: regulates menstruation, PMT
- *digestive*: tonifies liver and gall bladder.

When shouldn't it be used?
During pregnancy.

If you remember only one thing...
Carrot seed, like the vegetable of the same name, clears out the digestion and cleans up the skin.

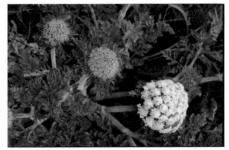

Chamomile (German)

This type is now known as blue chamomile.

What is its botanical name?
Matricaria recutica or *matricaria chamomilla*.

Where in the world does it come from?
Europe, specifically Hungary and Bulgaria although it is still grown and exported from Germany.

Which part of the plant is used to make the oil?
The flowers.

How is it extracted?
Steam distillation.

What is its chemical make-up?
German chamomile contains about 7% chamazulene (which is a product of the distillation process but does not exist in the flower), a T-erpene, and farnesol, an Al-Cohol. Its chemical make-up is T-AC.

What are its therapeutic actions?
German chamomile is
- analgesic
- anti-allergic
- anti-inflammatory
- antispasmodic
- emmenagogue (mild)

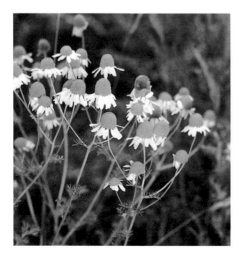

- sedative (nervous system)
- stimulant (immune system)
- vulnerary
- vermifuge.

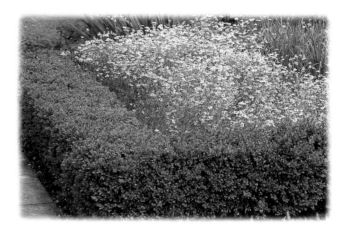

Which conditions/systems benefit from its use?
- *skin*: calms and soothes many skin conditions, especially allergies, bruises, eczema, blisters, acne, psoriasis and ulcers
- *skeletal*: eases aching joints and toothache
- *muscular*: relieves muscular pain in lower back
- *nervous*: relaxes thus relieving anxiety, tension and insomnia
- *reproductive*: antispasmodic so relieves period pain; also relieves symptoms of PMT and menopause
- *digestive*: regulates peristalsis thus relieving irritable bowel syndrome; relieves indigestion and nausea
- *immune*: stimulates whole system.

When shouldn't it be used?
In the early stages of pregnancy. Some very sensitive skins may react to it so a skin test should be used for testing reaction.

If you remember only one thing...
Chamomile is very versatile, calming and relaxing, good for children (especially if hyperactive), the frail and the elderly.

Chamomile (Roman)

What is its botanical name?
Chamaemelum nobile and *anthemis nobilis*.

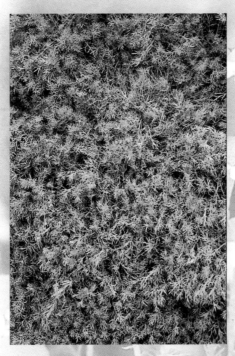

Where in the world does it come from?
Europe, especially England, Belgium, France and the USA.

Which part of the plant is used to make the oil?
The flowers.

How is the oil extracted?
By steam distillation.

What is its chemical make-up?
Roman chamomile is mostly angelic and tiglic acids (E-sters), isobutyl angelate (E-ster), pinocarvone (K-etone) and chamazulene (T-erpene). Its chemical make-up is thus E-AD-K-T.

What are its therapeutic actions?
Roman chamomile is

- analgesic
- anti-inflammatory
- antiseptic
- antispasmodic
- bactericidal
- emmenagogue
- sedative (nervous system)
- stomachic
- vulnerary
- vermifuge
- tonic.

Which conditions/systems benefit from its use?
- *skin*: rashes, allergies, dry skin conditions; effective for eczema, psoriasis
- *skeletal*: soothes joint inflammations, arthritis
- *muscular*: soothes inflammations, aches and pains
- *nervous*: stress, depression, insomnia, relaxing thus reduces tension and anxiety
- *digestive*: teeth abscesses, diarrhoea, nausea, upset stomach, nervous indigestion
- *reproductive*: premenstrual tension and fluid retention; relieves period pain and menopausal depression
- *urinary*: cystitis and other urinary tract infections.

When shouldn't it be used?
Roman chamomile should not be used during pregnancy but otherwise has no known contraindications and is good for use with children.

If you remember only one thing...
Roman chamomile, like the German variety, is calming and effective and a good all-round oil.

Clary sage

What is its botanical name?
Salvia sclarea.

Where in the world does it come from?
England, Russia, Morocco, France, Italy, Spain.

Which part of the plant is used to make the oil?
The leaves and flowers.

How is it extracted?
Steam distillation.

What is its chemical make-up?
Clary sage is mostly linalyl acetate (E-ster), linalol (Al-Cohol) and T-erpenes such as pinene and myrcene. Its chemical make-up is E-AC-T.

What are its therapeutic actions?
Clary sage is
- anti-inflammatory
- antispasmodic
- relaxing
- sedative
- tonic
- hypotensive oil and uplifting (only for the mind).

Which conditions/systems benefit from its use?
- *skin*: reduces inflammations
- *skeletal*: eases painful joints
- *muscular*: relaxes muscles, reduces spasm, muscle fatigue, cramp, fibrositis
- *nervous*: uplifts and promotes feeling of well-being/euphoria, soothes nervous tension, panic and acts as a sedative, relieves headache and migraine symptoms
- *reproductive/endocrine*: balances hormones, relieves PMT, fluid retention and painful cramps

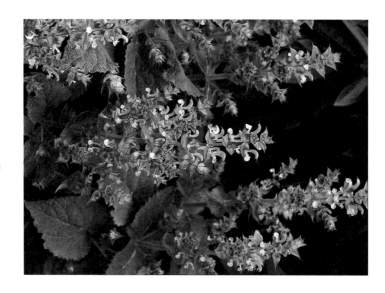

- *immune*: strengthens the immune system making it useful for the weak/convalescent.

When shouldn't it be used?
During pregnancy and before or after drinking alcohol (the oil can increase the effects of drunkenness).

If you remember only one thing...
Clary sage is warming, relaxing and uplifting.

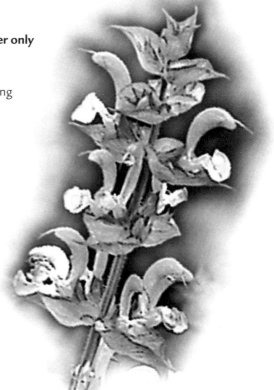

Coriander

A strong aromatic herb often used for children's digestive upsets and griping pains.

What is its botanical name?
Coriandrum sativum.

Where in the world does it come from?
Russia, Europe and Western Asia

Which part of the plant is used to make the oil?
Seeds.

How is it extracted?
Steam distillation.

What is its chemical make-up?
Coriander is mostly linalol and borneol (Al-Cohols) and decyl aldehyde (Al-Dehyde). Its chemical make-up is AD-AC.

What are its therapeutic actions?
Coriander is
- analgesic
- antispasmodic
- bactericidal
- depurative
- fungicidal
- stimulant
- uplifting.

Which conditions/systems benefit from its use?
- *circulation, muscles and joints*: arthritis, gout, muscular aches and pains, poor circulation, rheumatism and stiffness
- *digestive*: colic, nausea and spasm
- *immune system*: colds, flu and general infections
- *nervous system*: migraines and nervous exhaustion.

When shouldn't it be used?
Coriander should be used in moderation.

If you remember only one thing...
Coriander clears the mind and uplifts, helps to relieve headaches and migraines.

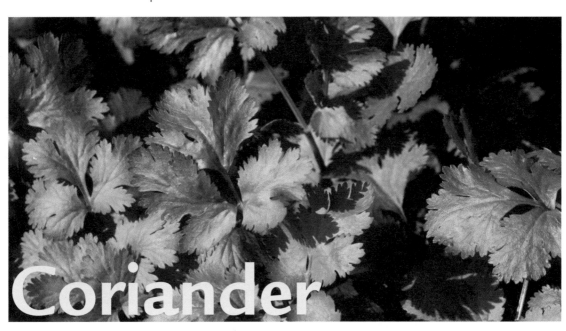

Coriander

Cypress

What is its botanical name?
Cupressus sempervirens.

Where in the world does it come from?
Mediterranean countries such as France, Spain, Italy, Portugal; also parts of North Africa.

Which part of the plant is used to make the oil?
Leaves and cones (like small fruits).

How is it extracted?
Steam distillation.

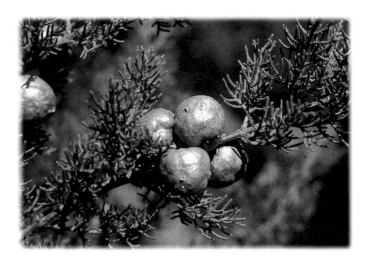

What is its chemical make-up?
Cypress is mainly T-erpenes (pinene and camphene) plus other trace molecules like sabinol (Al-Cohol). Its chemical make-up is T-AC.

What are its therapeutic actions?
Cypress is
- antispasmodic
- astringent
- depurative
- haemostatic
- diuretic
- tonic
- uplifting
- vasoconstrictive.

Which conditions/systems benefit from its use?
- *cells and tissues of whole body*: astringent; acts as a diuretic, acts on cellulite and water retention
- *skin*: controls water loss, oil and sweat production; good for sweaty, oily and mature skins
- *circulatory*: narrows blood vessels so eases varicose veins, haemorrhoids and heavy bleeding

- *reproductive*: regulates problems related to menstruation (heavy periods, PMT, hormonal and menopausal problems).

When shouldn't it be used?
Generally safe and non-irritating though it is not recommended for use during pregnancy.

If you remember only one thing...
Cypress is a strong astringent and depurative so it controls the body's production of liquids (excess sweat or oil, fluid retention, heavy menstrual bleeding).

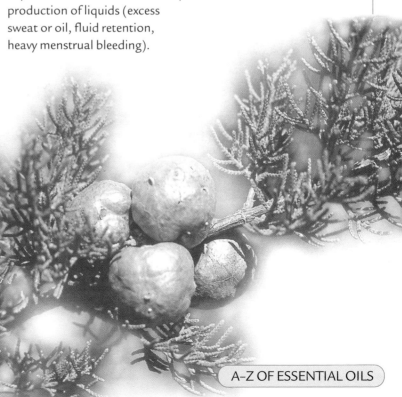

Eucalyptus (blue gum)

There are several types of eucalyptus so check the botanical name of the oil purchased/used to ensure it is the one you want. The type which is used the most in aromatherapy is blue gum, the common species.

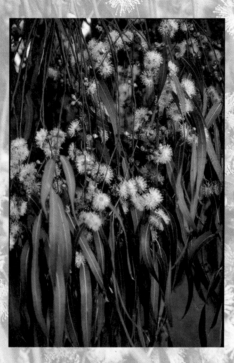

What is its botanical name?
Eucalyptus globulus.

Where in the world does it come from?
The eucalyptus tree is a native of Tasmania and Australia but it is now grown in Mediterranean countries like Spain and Portugal.

Which part of the plant is used to make the oil?
The leaves and twigs of the tree.

How is it extracted?
Steam distillation.

What is its chemical make-up?
Eucalyptus is mostly cineol (O-xide) and T-erpenes such as limonene and pinene. Its chemical make-up is O-T.

What are its therapeutic actions?
Eucalyptus (blue gum) is
- analgesic
- antiseptic
- antispasmodic
- antiviral
- depurative
- expectorant
- prophylactic
- stimulant
- uplifting.

Which conditions/systems benefit from its use?
- *skin*: infections and dull, congested skin, burns, wounds, outbreaks of spots
- *skeletal*: eases rheumatism
- *muscular*: relieves aches and pains
- *nervous system*: clears the head, calms emotions
- *respiratory*: effective for all cold and flu symptoms as well as throat infections, catarrh, sinusitis, asthma, infections, coughs (expectorant – clears mucus by encouraging coughs)
- *urinary*: cystitis
- *immune*: stimulates body's immunity against infection.

When shouldn't it be used?
Eucalyptus should only be used in low dilutions since it may irritate the skin. It is incompatible with homeopathic treatments.

If you remember only one thing...
Eucalyptus protects the whole body against disease and viruses by strengthening the immune system.

● **Did you know?**

Eucalyptus is used in many cold and flu remedies.

Fennel

It is important to distinguish between sweet fennel and bitter fennel. Sweet fennel is widely used in aromatherapy but bitter fennel is considered too toxic.

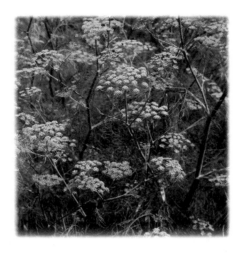

What is its botanical name?
Foeniculum vulgare var. *dulce*.

Where in the world does it come from?
Mediterranean countries such as France, Italy and Greece.

Which part of the plant is used to make the oil?
The crushed seeds.

How is it extracted?
Steam distillation.

What is its chemical make-up?
Sweet fennel is mostly anethole (P-henol) and limonene, pinene and phellandrene (T-erpenes) plus traces of other molecules. Its chemical make-up is P-T.

What are its therapeutic actions?
Sweet fennel is
- antiseptic
- antispasmodic
- carminative
- depurative
- galactagogue
- emmenagogue
- laxative
- antimicrobial
- tonic.

Which conditions/ systems benefit from its use?
- *skin*: clears congestion; antiseptic qualities help bruises to heal and relieve pain and irritation from bites and stings
- *skeletal*: helps rheumatism
- *circulatory*: helps reduce cellulite
- *nervous*: gives a sense of strength and courage
- *digestive*: cleans out intestines, liver, colon; relieves colic, flatulence, constipation
- *reproductive*: eases PMT, amenorrhoea and menopausal problems; increases milk flow in nursing mothers
- *urinary*: cleanses kidneys and stimulates them
- *general*: detoxifies the body; good for hangovers.

When shouldn't it be used?
During pregnancy, for epileptics and in large doses (which can be narcotic). Otherwise, it is generally non-toxic and safe to use on the skin.
NB Sweet fennel should never be confused with bitter fennel which is not recommended for use.

If you remember only one thing...
Fennel cleans out the body. It is a natural diuretic and depurative, so it helps to get rid of cellulite, flatulence, water retention or constipation.

Did you know?
Sweet fennel is one of the main ingredients in babies' gripe water.

Frankincense

What is its botanical name?
Boswellia carteri.

Where in the world does it come from?
Frankincense, as might be obvious from its Biblical associations, comes from a tree or shrub which grows in the Red Sea region. It now also grows in Africa, especially the north-east, Somalia and Ethiopia.

Which part of the plant is used to make the oil?
The resin of the tree or shrub.

How is it extracted?
Steam distillation.

What is its chemical make-up?
Frankincense is mostly pinene and limonene (T-erpenes) plus trace molecules. Its chemical make-up is T.

What are its therapeutic actions?
Frankincense is

- expectorant
- haemostatic
- relaxing
- rubefacient
- sedative
- tonic
- vermifuge.

Which conditions/systems benefit from its use?

- *skin*: rejuvenates mature skins by smoothing wrinkles and dry skins; balances oily skins
- *nervous*: comforting, warming, relaxing; burn (in a burner) during meditation to help focus the mind
- *respiratory*: helps asthma, bronchitis, coughs, laryngitis; clears mucus and catarrh; calms breathing
- *urinary*: eases symptoms of cystitis, nephritis and genital infections.

When shouldn't it be used?
Frankincense is non-toxic and non-irritant.

If you remember only one thing...
Frankincense is emotionally balancing, producing a sense of calm.

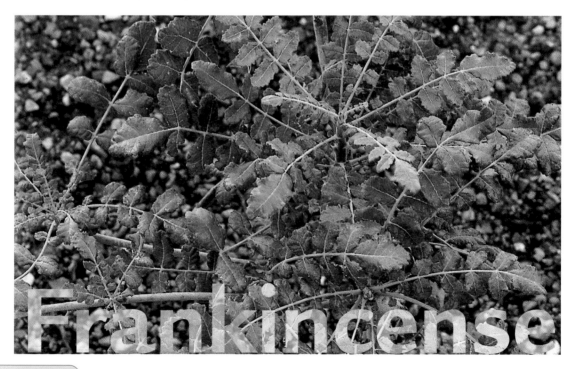

Frankincense

Geranium

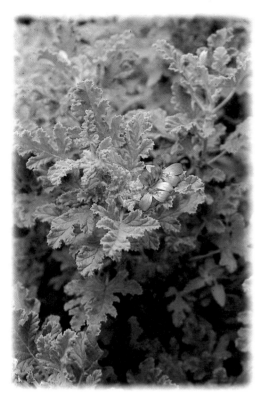

What is its botanical name?
Pelargonium graveolens or *pelargonium odoratissimum*.

Where in the world does it come from?
Geranium plants are originally natives of South Africa but are now grown worldwide, especially in Mediterranean Europe, Russia and Egypt.

Which part of the plant is used to make the oil?
The whole plant contains the essential oil so most of it is used: the leaves, flowers and flower stalks.

How is it extracted?
Steam distillation.

What is its chemical make-up?
Geranium is mostly geraniol and citronellol (Al-Cohols) with traces of limonene (T-erpene) and menthone (K-etone). Its chemical make-up is AC-T-K.

What are its therapeutic actions?
Geranium is
- diuretic
- anti-inflammatory
- balancing
- haemostatic
- vulnerary
- vermifuge
- stimulant
- tonic
- uplifting.

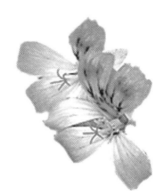

Which conditions/systems benefit from its use?
- *skin*: benefits all skin types, balances sebum, helps keep skin supple, tonifies dull, congested skins, improves circulation thus preventing chilblains and enlivening pale skin
- *circulatory/lymphatic*: improves circulation and stimulates lymphatic system
- *nervous*: tonic, lifts the spirits and relieves anxiety, depression and stress
- *endocrine/reproductive*: balances the hormones, thus regulating PMT, menopause (especially the depression associated with this), and heavy periods.

When shouldn't it be used?
On very sensitive skin. Otherwise it is completely safe.

If you remember only one thing...
Geranium balances both mind and body, is emotionally uplifting and stimulates the circulation.

Ginger

What is its botanical name?
Zingiber officinale.

Where in the world does it come from?
Asia (especially India), tropical countries (especially Jamaica and the West Indies) and Nigeria.

Which part of the plant is used to make the oil?
The thick, horizontal root of the plant, known as a rhizome.

How is it extracted?
By steam distillation.

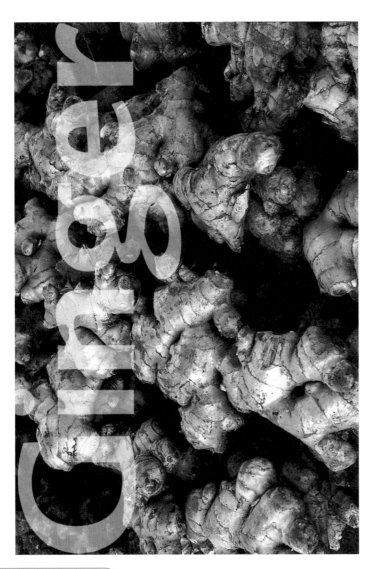

What is its chemical make-up?
Zingiberene (S-esquiterpene), gingerol (Al-Cohol) and gingerone (K-etone) plus traces of Terpenes like camphene, other alcohols and citronellal (Al-Dehyde). Its chemical make-up is S-T-AC-K-AD.

What are its therapeutic actions?
Ginger is
- stimulating
- tonic
- analgesic
- laxative
- warming.

Which conditions/systems benefit from its use?
- *skin*: stimulates circulation thus helps heal bruises and chilblains
- *skeletal*: eases joint pain, arthritis and rheumatoid arthritis
- *muscular*: relieves cramps, muscle spasms and sprains
- *circulatory*: stimulates the circulation which helps to ease blood vessel problems such as varicose veins
- *nervous*: warms emotions, especially when lethargic and fatigued, heightens senses and improves memory
- *digestive*: settles the stomach, nausea, motion sickness, stimulates appetite
- *respiratory*: eases flu and cold symptoms, especially catarrh, sore throats, fever, runny nose
- *general*: removes toxins, stimulates and wakes up body.

When shouldn't it be used?
On very sensitive skins as it can be phototoxic. Ginger is spicy and can thus be an irritant. It should only be used in low concentrations.

If you remember only one thing...
Ginger is spicy and warm. It stimulates the circulation and wakes up sluggish, tired bodies. It also calms and settles the stomach.

Grapefruit

What is its botanical name?
Citrus paradisi.

Where in the world does it come from?
Tropical Asia, the West Indies, California.

Which part of the plant is used to make the oil?
The fruit peel.

How is it extracted?
Expression.

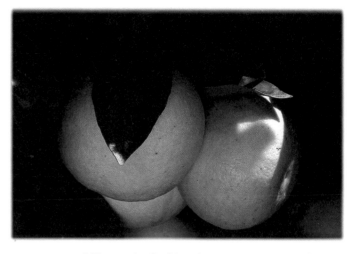

What is its chemical make-up?
Grapefruit is 90% limonene (T-erpene), plus cadinene (also a T-erpene), paradisiol (Al-Cohol), neral (Al-Dehyde) and other trace molecules. Its chemical make-up is T-AC-AD.

What are its therapeutic actions?
Grapefruit is
- astringent
- depurative
- diuretic
- stimulant
- tonic
- uplifting.

Which conditions/systems benefit from its use?
- *skin*: astringent for dull, oily skin and acne
- *lymphatic*: diuretic thus reduces water retention and oedemas, helps cellulite
- *nervous*: uplifting and refreshing thus revives depressed and stressed minds, creates euphoric feeling and balances mood swings
- *immune*: stimulates immunity and helps to prevent colds and flu
- *general*: fatigue, jet-lag, morning tiredness.

When shouldn't it be used?
Grapefruit is safe and not an irritant. Also, unlike other citrus oils, it is only phototoxic when distilled. However, if the extraction method is not known it should be treated as phototoxic.

If you remember only one thing...
Grapefruit is a refreshing tonic and has an uplifting effect, thus helps combat depression (especially S.A.D.), lethargy and general fatigue.

Grapefruit

Jasmine

What is its botanical name?
Jasminum officinale.

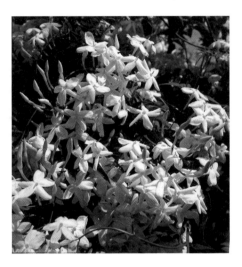

Where in the world does it come from?
China, northern India, Egypt, France and many Mediterranean countries.

Which part of the plant is used to make the oil?
The flowers.

How is it extracted?
Solvent extraction which produces an absolute, which is then steam distilled. The traditional method (and the most expensive) is enfleurage.

What is its chemical make-up?
Jasmine is mostly benzyl acetate (E-ster) and linalol (Al-Cohol) plus many others including jasmone (K-etone). Its chemical make-up is E-AC-K.

What are its therapeutic actions?
Jasmine is
- antispasmodic
- galactagogue
- relaxing
- sedative
- tonic
- tonic (uterine).

Which conditions/systems benefit from its use?
- *skin*: encourages cell renewal thus heals scar tissues and reduces stretch marks; hydrates and soothes dry, mature skin and increases elasticity
- *nervous*: improves self-confidence, optimism, lifts depression, calms nerves and warms emotions; eases nerve pain
- *reproductive/endocrine*: balances hormones in PMT and menopause; eases child labour pains and speeds up delivery.

When shouldn't it be used?
Jasmine is useful at the end of pregnancy, because it strengthens uterine contractions, but it is thus not recommended for use during pregnancy.

If you remember only one thing...
Jasmine rejuvenates the skin and the soul, relaxes, soothes and uplifts.

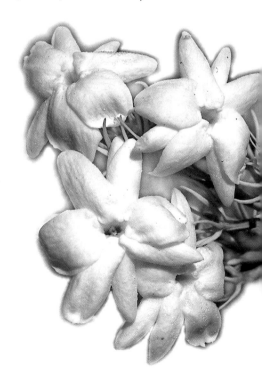

Juniper (berry)

What is its botanical name?

Juniperus communis.

Where in the world does it come from?

Juniper naturally grows in the north, particularly Siberia, Canada and in Scandinavian countries. However, the oil is mainly produced in France, Italy, Hungary, the Czech Republic and Slovakia.

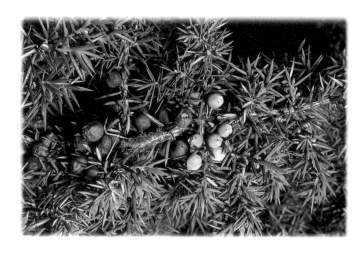

Which part of the plant is used to make the oil?

The best oil comes from the dried berries but a cheaper oil is made from the needles and wood of the tree.

NB Only juniper berry oil is recommended for use in aromatherapy.

How is it extracted?

By steam distillation.

What is its chemical make-up?

Juniper is mainly T-erpenes, especially pinene, myrcene and sabinene. Its chemical make-up is thus T.

What are its therapeutic actions?

Juniper is

- analgesic
- antiseptic
- antispasmodic
- depurative
- diuretic
- relaxing
- sedative
- stimulant
- tonic
- warming.

Which conditions/systems benefit from its use?

- *skin*: detoxifies blocked pores, acne, oily skin; good for dermatitis, psoriasis and eczema

- *skeletal*: warming effect eases symptoms of arthritis, rheumatism and gout
- *circulatory*: aids cellulite
- *nervous*: clears and stimulates the mind, relieves stress-related conditions and tension
- *urinary*: cystitis; diuretic helps fluid retention.

When shouldn't it be used?

Juniper is an abortifacient (stimulates the uterus muscles) so it should never be used during pregnancy. It may also irritate the kidneys and should not be used on those with kidney disease or on those who have ever suffered from nephritis. Prolonged use can cause kidney damage.

If you remember only one thing...

Juniper detoxifies, cleaning out the body and mind of excesses, whether fluids, anxieties or the build-up of toxins.

> **Did you know?** ●
>
> **Gin gets its flavour from juniper berries.**

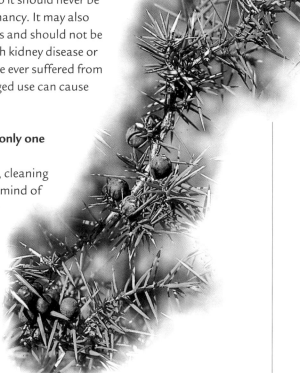

Lavender (true)

Lavender is a good oil to learn with because it is very versatile and not very expensive.

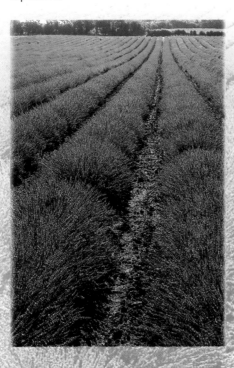

What is its botanical name?
Lavandula angustifolia and *lavandula officinalis.*

Where in the world does it come from?
Mediterranean countries, especially France, and England.

Which part of the plant is used to make the oil?
The flowers.

How is it extracted?
By steam distillation.

What is its chemical make-up?
Lavender has too many constituents to list (more than 100). However, the main ones are linalyl acetate and lavandulyl acetate (E-sters) plus linalol and lavandulol (Al-Cohols) Its chemical make-up is E-AC.

What are its therapeutic actions?
Lavender is
- analgesic
- anti-inflammatory
- antiseptic
- antispasmodic
- antiviral
- balancing
- cooling
- detoxifying
- fungicidal
- relaxing
- sedative
- tonic
- uplifting.

Which conditions/systems benefit from its use?
skin: effective for use on all skin types and conditions – balances sebum in oily skin, promotes cell growth and rapid healing for scars and stretch marks, antiseptic for insect bites and stings, burns, sunburns, wounds, healing for dermatitis and psoriasis
skeletal: eases rheumatism
muscular: soothes and relieves aches and sprains
circulatory: lowers high blood pressure and other stress-related conditions such as palpitations
nervous: balances emotions, lifts depression, relieves stress, insomnia and anxiety; relieves headaches, migraine, tension, shock
respiratory: relaxes breathing, eases bronchitis, laryngitis; antiviral effect on flu and colds.

When shouldn't it be used?
Lavender is neither toxic nor irritating.

If you remember only one thing...
The whole body can benefit from lavender. It is an all-rounder, useful for treating all conditions as well as relaxing and balancing the whole body.

Lemon

What is its botanical name?
Citrus limon.

Where in the world does it come from?
Lemon trees are cultivated all over the world. They are native to Asia and India and also grow wild in Mediterranean countries such as Spain and Portugal.

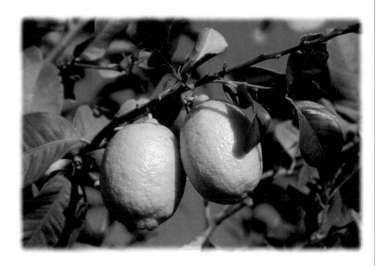

Which part of the plant is used to make the oil?
The fresh peel (zest) of the fruit.

How is it extracted?
Expression.

What is its chemical make-up?
Lemon is mostly limonene and pinene (T-erpenes) plus citronellol (Al-Cohol) and citral (Al-Dehyde). Its chemical make-up is T-AC-AD.

What are its therapeutic actions?
Lemon is
- anti-acid
- antiseptic
- antiviral
- detoxifying
- fungicidal
- haemostatic
- stimulant
- tonic
- uplifting.

Which conditions/systems benefit from its use?
- *skin*: useful for boils, warts, acne/other seborrhoeic conditions
- *circulatory*: tonifies blood and improves circulation, reduces pressure on varicose veins, lowers high blood pressure, slows external bleeding including nosebleeds
- *nervous*: refreshes and stimulates the mind, allowing clarity of thought
- *digestive*: though high in citric acid, lemon actually reduces the high levels of gastric acid which cause ulcers; dyspepsia
- *respiratory*: protects against infections like colds and flu, lowers temperature
- *immune*: stimulates immune system to produce protective white blood cells.

When shouldn't it be used?
Lemon oil is phototoxic and may cause sensitivity to sunlight. It may irritate skin and should thus be used in low concentrations.

If you remember only one thing...
Lemon protects and stimulates the body's systems and lifts the emotions.

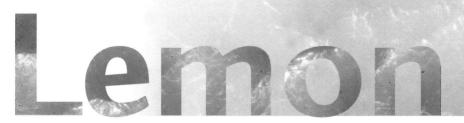

Lemongrass

Lemongrass is an important ingredient in Thai cuisine, and the oil, like the plant has a lemony and spicy quality.

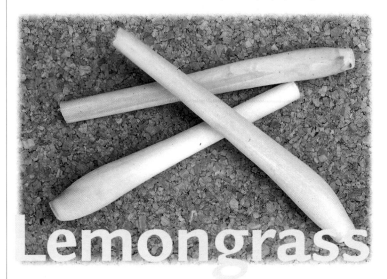

What is its botanical name?
Cymbopogon citratus.

Where in the world does it come from?
Lemongrass grows in Asia, in the West Indies and East India.

Which part of the plant is used to make the oil?
The leaves of the grass (both fresh and part-dried).

How is it extracted?
By steam distillation.

What is its chemical make-up?
Lemongrass is mostly citral (Al-Dehyde), geraniol (Al-Cohol) plus traces of other molecules such as limonene and myrcene (T-erpenes). Its chemical make-up is AD-AC-T.

What are its therapeutic actions?
Lemongrass is
- antidepressant
- antiseptic
- astringent
- stimulant
- tonic
- uplifting.

Which conditions/systems benefit from its use?
- *skin*: tonifies open pores, acne, oily skin; insect-repellent
- *skeletal*: useful for aching joints, gout, rheumatism
- *muscular*: tonifies aching muscles, tired legs and veins, relieves muscle fatigue; useful for sports injuries
- *nervous*: stimulates, revives, energises the emotions and relieves stress-related conditions and nervous exhaustion
- *digestive*: stimulates appetite, relieves indigestion and gastro-enteritis
- *respiratory*: antiseptic effect on infections, sore throats, laryngitis
- *immune system*: reduces fever.

When shouldn't it be used?
Lemongrass is non-toxic but may irritate the skin.

If you remember only one thing...
Lemongrass is refreshing and stimulating for muscles and skin.

Lime

The fruit is often used in place of lemon with which it shares many qualities, and is used for similar purposes including infections, sore throats, cold etc.

What is its botanical name?
Citrus Medica.

Where in the world does it come from?
Originally from Asia, cultivated in many warm places Italy, West Indies and the Americas.

Which part of the plant is used to make the oil?
The peel and the whole fruit

How is it extracted?
Expression/Steam distillation.

What is its chemical make-up?
Lime is mostly made up of Limonene and pinene (T-erpenes). Its chemical make-up is T

What are its therapeutic actions?
Lime is
- antiseptic
- antiviral
- astringent
- tonic
- febrifuge
- uplifting
- hypotensive.

Which conditions/systems benefit from its use?
- *skin*: Acne, boils, oily skin and warts
- *circulatory*: Tonifies blood and improves circulation, cellulite, lowers high blood pressure, slows external bleeding including nose bleeds
- *nervous*: Uplifting, ideal for fatigue and tired minds
- *digestive*: Dyspepsia
- *respiratory*: Colds, flu and infections, lowers temperature
- *immune*: Stimulates immune system.

When shouldn't it be used?
Expressed peel is photo-toxic but not the steam distilled oil

If you remember only one thing...
Lime is very stimulating and activating especially where there is apathy, anxiety and depression.

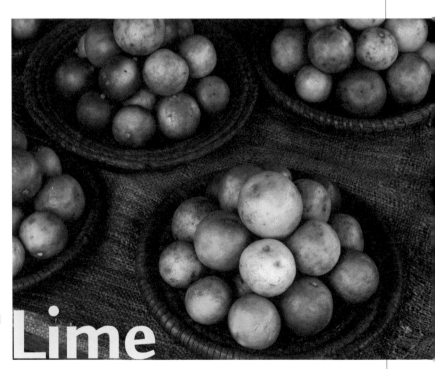

Lime

Mandarin

Mandarin is a member of the citrus family. It is known as tangerine in North America.

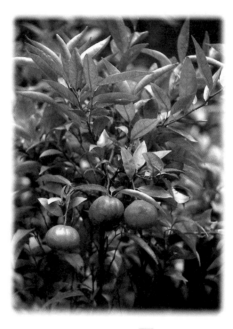

What is its botanical name?
Citrus reticulata.

Where in the world does it come from?
Southern China and Eastern Asia.

Which part of the plant is used to make the oil?
The peel of the fruit.

How is it extracted?
Expression.

What is its chemical make-up?
Like other citrus fruits, limonene (T-erpene) is the main constituent plus methyl methylanthranilate (E-ster), geraniol (Al-Cohol) and citral (Al-Dehyde). Its chemical make-up is T-E-AC-AD.

What are its therapeutic actions?
Mandarin is
- antiviral
- carminative
- relaxing
- antispasmodic
- tonic
- sedative
- uplifting.

Which conditions/systems benefit from its use?
- *skin*: helps cell growth for scar tissue and stretch marks; astringent for oily skin
- *lymphatic*: mild diuretic qualities help cellulite
- *nervous*: mandarin's refreshing aroma lifts anxiety and symptoms of depression as well as helping insomniacs
- *reproductive*: helps PMT
- *digestive*: tonifies digestion, expels wind, calms the stomach and stimulates appetite.

When shouldn't it be used?
It can be mildly phototoxic if used before exposure to sunlight.

If you remember only one thing…
Mandarin is refreshing and happy, soothing and relaxing and eases all aspects of nervous exhaustion and anxiety. It is useful for treating children and the frail or elderly and is the only oil considered safe for use after the first trimester of pregnancy.

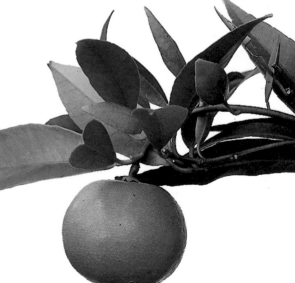

Marjoram (sweet)

What is its botanical name?
Origanum majorana.

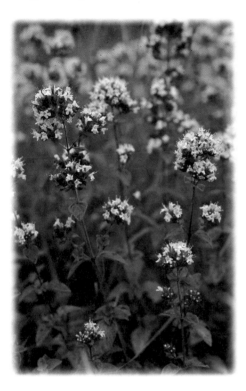

Where in the world does it come from?
Mediterranean countries such as Spain, France and Egypt; also parts of North Africa.

Which part of the plant is used to make the oil?
Dried flowers and leaves.

How is it extracted?
By steam distillation.

What is its chemical make-up?
Marjoram contains terpineol, linalol (Al-Cohols), terpinene and sabinene (T-erpenes) plus geranyl acetate and linalyl acetate (E-sters). Its chemical make-up is AC-T-E.

What are its therapeutic actions?
Marjoram is
- analgesic
- antispasmodic
- emmenagogue
- relaxing
- sedative
- tonic
- nervine
- laxative
- vulnerary
- vasodilatory
- warming.

Which conditions/systems benefit from its use?
- *skin*: helps heal bruises
- *skeletal*: eases joint problems
- *muscular*: eases aches and pains, especially after sport, also helps period cramps
- *circulatory*: lowers high blood pressure, improves poor circulation and prevents chilblains
- *nervous*: calms and soothes the emotions, especially in times of stress, grief and loneliness; good for headaches, insomnia and migraines
- *digestive*: eases stomach cramps, indigestion and constipation
- *respiratory*: eases congestion in nose and sinuses, relieves asthma and bronchitis.

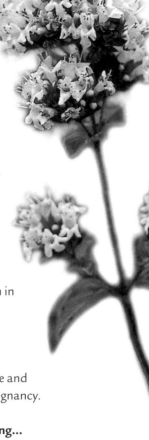

When shouldn't it be used?
Marjoram is an emmenagogue and should not be used during pregnancy.

If you remember only one thing...
Marjoram is a soothing and comforting oil, which calms over-active minds, warms the body and relieves anxiety and distress.

Melissa (lemon balm)

What is its botanical name?
Melissa officinalis.

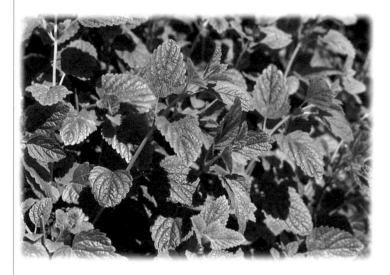

Where does it come from?
Mediterranean countries such as France and Spain and Germany.

Which part of the plant is used to make the oil?
The leaves and flowers of the herb.

How is it extracted?
By steam distillation.

What is its chemical make-up?
Melissa is mostly citral (Al-Dehyde) and Al-Cohols (geraniol and citronellol). Its chemical make-up is AD-AC.

What are its therapeutic actions?
Melissa is
- anti-allergic
- anti-inflammatory
- antispasmodic
- antiviral
- cooling
- emmenagogue
- relaxing
- sedative
- tonic
- vermifuge
- nervine
- uplifting.

Which conditions/systems benefit from its use?
- *skin*: anti-allergic so prevents/soothes allergic reactions and problems such as dermatitis and eczema; insect bites and stings
- *circulatory*: reduces high blood pressure and slows down the heartbeat
- *nervous*: reduces anxiety and depression, calms nerves
- *reproductive*: eases depression associated with PMT and menopause; helps regulate menstruation.

When shouldn't it be used?
Melissa provokes menstruation so should be avoided during pregnancy. It is also generally used in weak dilutions.
NB Unless absolutely sure of the source, it should be avoided since there are many other cheaper oils with similar properties.

If you remember only one thing...
Melissa is uplifting and extremely good for stress-related conditions and shock.

Melissa

Myrrh

What is its botanical name?
Commiphora myrrha.

Where in the world does it come from?
Red Sea area and North-east Africa
(Ethiopia, Sudan); South-west Asia.

Which part of the plant is used to make the oil?
The resin of the myrrh shrub or tree.

How is it extracted?
A resinoid is extracted by solvent
extraction and an essential oil by steam
distillation.

What is its chemical make-up?
Myrrh is mostly heerabolene and
limonene (T-erpenes), and
cinnamaldehyde (Al-Dehyde). Its
chemical make-up is T-AC-AD.

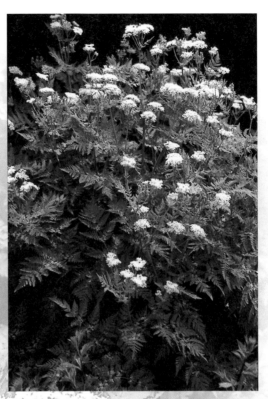

What are its therapeutic actions?
Myrrh is
- anticatarrhal
- anti-inflammatory
- antiseptic
- carminative
- cicatrisant
- cooling
- emmenagogue
- expectorant
- fungicidal
- sedative
- vulnerary
- stimulant (digestive, pulmonary)
- tonic.

Which conditions/systems benefit from its use?
- *skin*: chapped skin, fungus infections
  like athlete's foot and ringworm,
  wounds; good for mature skins
- *nervous*: stimulates and revives,
  relieving apathy, lack of motivation
  and general lethargy
- *reproductive*: regulates menstrual cycle;

relieves thrush
- *digestive*: mouth and gum ulcers,
  gingivitis; stimulates appetite, aids
  diarrhoea, flatulence
- *respiratory*: myrrh is good for helping
  all respiratory problems; anticatarrhal
  and expectorant thus helps remove
  mucus from lungs; antiseptic and anti-
  inflammatory thus good for all
  infections, colds, bronchitis and
  glandular fever.

When shouldn't it be used?
Myrrh is not recommended for use
during pregnancy or in high
concentration.
*NB It takes more than 24 hours to eliminate
myrrh from the body and thus it should not be
used on a regular or prolonged basis.*

If you remember only one thing...
Myrrh is a healer, especially good for
healing wounds, mouth and gum
problems and infections of the
respiratory system.

Neroli (Orange blossom)

What is its botanical name?

Citrus aurantium var. *amara* and *neroli bigarade*.

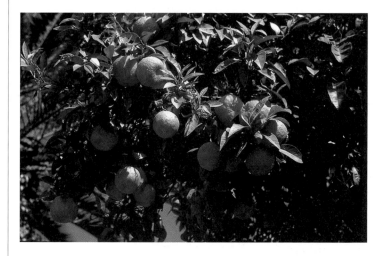

Where in the world does it come from?

Mediterranean countries (Italy, France, Spain), parts of North Africa and China.

Which part of the plant is used to make the oil?

Orange blossom flowers.

How is it extracted?

Solvent extraction or steam distillation.

What is its chemical make-up?

Neroli is mostly linalol (34% – Al-Cohol), limonene (T-erpene) and linalyl acetate (6-17% – E-ster). Its chemical make-up is AC-T-E.

What are its therapeutic actions?

Neroli is

- antidepressant
- antispasmodic
- antiviral
- detoxifying
- relaxing
- sedative
- tonic
- uplifting.

Which conditions/systems benefit from its use?

- *skin*: helps cell regeneration (tonic) thus benefiting dry, mature skins, scars and stretch marks, thread veins, eczema and psoriasis
- *circulatory*: tonic for circulation (especially varicose veins) and eases palpitations (due to calming effect)
- *nervous*: lifts depression, relieves stress-related conditions, especially insomnia, and anxiety; eases neuralgia, calms and soothes nerves and nerve endings
- *reproductive*: relieves PMT.

When shouldn't it be used?

Neroli is not known to have any contraindications.

If you remember only one thing...

Neroli is a positive thinker, helping to boost confidence and self-esteem and reducing negative emotions. It rejuvenates body and soul!

Neroli

Niaouli

An oil that is used generally for aches and pains and infections.

What is its botanical name?
Melaleuca viridiflora.

Where in the world does it come from?
Australia and Tasmania.

Which part of the plant is used to make the oil?
Leaves and young twigs.

How is it extracted?
Steam distillation.

What is its chemical make-up?
Niaouli is mostly cineole (O-xide) and terpineol (Al-Cohols). Its chemical make-up is O–AC

What are its therapeutic actions?
Niaouli is
- analgesic
- antiseptic
- expectorant
- bactericidal
- cicatrisant
- stimulant

Which conditions/systems benefit from its use?
- *skin*: acne, boils, cuts, insect bites, oily skin
- *circulation, muscles and joints*: aches and pains, poor circulation and rheumatism
- *respiratory*: asthma, coughs and sinusitis, sore throats and whooping coughs
- *urinary*: cystitis and general urinary infections
- *immune*: colds and flu

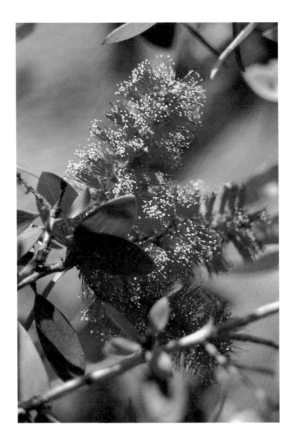

When shouldn't it be used?
Often subject to adulteration, non-toxic and non-irritant.

If you remember only one thing...
Niaouli is generally stimulating and uplifting, clears the head.

Orange (sweet)

What is its botanical name?
Citrus sinensis.

Where in the world does it come from?
The sweet orange is native to China but is extensively grown in California, Florida and Mediterranean countries (such as Spain, France, Italy).

Which part of the plant is used to make the oil?
The peel of the fruit.

How is it extracted?
Expression or steam distillation, but the distilled oil is a poorer quality and phototoxic.

What is its chemical make-up?
Sweet orange is mostly limonene (T-erpene). Its chemical make-up is T.

What are its therapeutic actions?
Sweet orange is
- antidepressant
- antispasmodic
- antiviral
- hypotensive
- sedative
- stimulant (digestive, lymphatic)
- stomachic
- uplifting
- sedative (nervous).

Which conditions/systems benefit from its use?
- *skin*: skin tonic for dull, oily skins; refreshes and detoxifies
- *circulatory*: hypotensive thus lowers blood pressure
- *lymphatic*: relieves oedema and fluid retention
- *nervous*: provokes positive outlook, refreshes the mind, lifts and relieves depression, tension and stress
- *digestive*: calms the stomach, aids peristalsis, helps relieve digestive problems such as diarrhoea and constipation
- *immune*: helps protect against infections, colds and flu.

When shouldn't it be used?
Expressed sweet orange oil is safe but the distilled version causes phototoxicity (sensitivity to sunlight).

If you remember only one thing...
Sweet orange is a member of the citrus family. These fruits only grow naturally in sunny hot countries and the oils from them are like a burst of sunshine: uplifting, warm, bright, restorative.

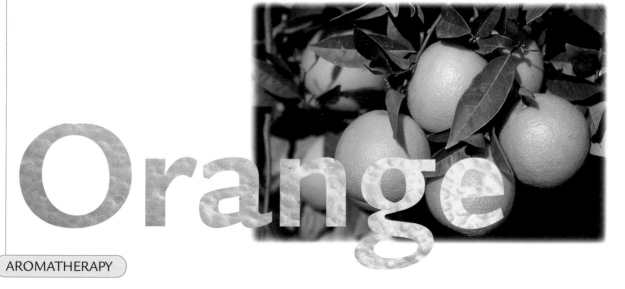

Orange

Palmarosa

What is its botanical name?
Cymbopogon martinii.

Where in the world does it come from?
Originally from India now cultivated in the Comoro Islands, Africa, Indonesia and Madagascar.

Which part of the plant is used to make the oil?
Fresh/dried grass.

How is it extracted?
Steam distillation.

What is its chemical make-up?
Palmarosa is mostly made up of Geraniol & Farnesol(AL-Cohol). Its chemical make-up is AC.

What are its therapeutic actions?
Palmarosa is
- antiseptic
- bactericidal
- cicatrisant
- febrifuge
- stimulant (digestive)
- tonic
- calming.

Which conditions/systems benefit from its use?
- *skin*: acne, minor skin infections, wrinkles, moisturises the skin, stimulates cellular regeneration and regulates sebum production
- *digestive*: intestinal infections and general digestive problems
- *nervous*: nervous exhaustion and stress related conditions.

When shouldn't it be used?
Palmarosa is non-toxic and non-irritant.

If you remember only one thing...
Palmarosa has a calming yet uplifting effect on emotions.

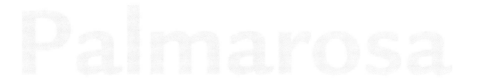

Patchouli

What is its botanical name?
Pogestemon cablin.

Where in the world does it come from?
Asia: Philippines, Indonesia, Malaysia, China, India.

Which part of the plant is used to make the oil?
The dried leaves.

How is it extracted?
Steam distillation.

What is its chemical make-up?
Patchouli is mostly patchouli alcohol and patchoulol (Al-Cohols) and patchoulene (T-erpene). Its chemical make-up is AC-T.

What are its therapeutic actions?
Patchouli is
- antidepressant
- anti-inflammatory
- cytophylactic
- diuretic
- fungicidal
- sedative
- stimulant
- tonic
- antimicrobial
- nervine
- prophylactic
- uplifting.

Which conditions/systems benefit from its use?
- *skin*: helps cell growth, scarred tissue, chapped skin; insect repellent
- *nervous system*: relieves stress-related conditions, lethargy, anxiety
- *digestive*: stimulant; helps peristalsis, aids weight loss.

When shouldn't it be used?
Patchouli should be used in low concentrations since it may cause phototoxicity.

If you remember only one thing...
Patchouli is both stimulant and sedative: a small amount stimulates the nervous and digestive systems; a large amount is relaxing and soothing.

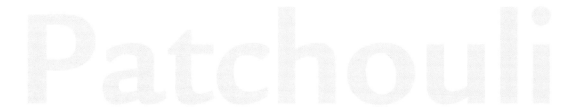

Peppermint

What is its botanical name?
Mentha piperita.

Where in the world does it come from?
English peppermint is the best but it is grown worldwide. Most peppermint oil now comes from the USA.

Which part of the plant is used to make the oil?
The leaves and flowers.

How is it extracted?
Steam distillation.

What is its chemical make-up?
Peppermint is mainly menthol (29-48% –Al-Cohol), menthone (20-31% – K-etone), menthyl acetate (E-ster), plus limonene (T-erpene) and pulegone (K-etone). Its chemical make-up is thus AC-K-E-T.

What are its therapeutic actions?
Peppermint is
- analgesic
- antiseptic
- antispasmodic
- antiviral
- antipruritic
- carminative
- cephalic
- cooling
- expectorant
- febrifuge
- stimulant
- stomachic
- tonic
- vermifuge
- uplifting
- vasoconstrictive.

Which conditions/systems benefit from its use?
- *skin*: vasoconstrictor thus reduces inflammations, itching; cooling effect on sunburn, hot flushes
- *nervous*: wakes up and refreshes the mind, improves concentration, helps mental fatigue, headaches and depression; cools and calms anger, hysteria, nervous trembling
- *digestive*: effective for flatulence, indigestion, nausea, travel sickness
- *respiratory*: decongests blocked sinuses, relieves asthma, cold and flu symptoms; encourages perspiration thus reducing fever
- *general*: relieves pain and cools – head-aches, migraines, toothache, aching feet.

When shouldn't it be used?
Peppermint counteracts the benefits of homeopathic remedies and should not be used with, or even stored near them. It should also be avoided late in the day and by insomniacs since it refreshes the mind, waking you up!

If you remember only one thing…
Peppermint is cool, refreshing and good for the digestion.

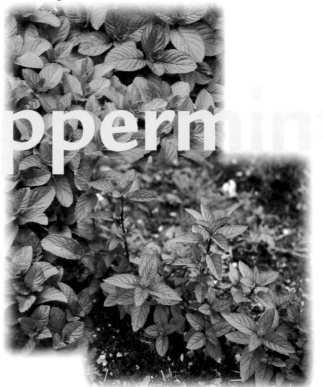

Petitgrain

What is its botanical name?
Citrus aurantium var. *amara*.

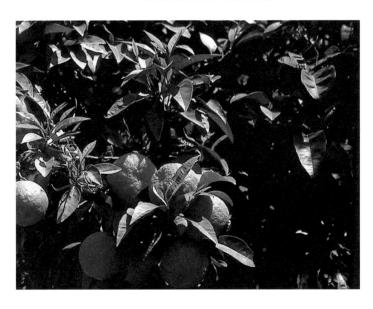

Where in the world does it come from?
Mediterranean countries, especially
France, parts of North Africa; Paraguay.

Which part of the plant is used to make the oil?
The leaves and twigs.

How is it extracted?
By steam distillation.

What is its chemical make-up?
Petitgrain is mostly linalyl acetate and
geranyl acetate (E-sters), plus Al-Cohols
(linalol, nerol, terpineol, geraniol). Its
chemical make-up is E-AC.

What are its therapeutic actions?
Petitgrain is
- antidepressant
- antiseptic
- antispasmodic
- digestive
- relaxing
- stimulant (digestive, nervous)
- nervine
- tonic
- uplifting.

Which conditions/systems benefit from its use?
- *skin*: tonic for greasy skin and hair
- *nervous*: soothes anxiety, tension,
  hyper-activity; sedates nervous spasms
  and physical problems relating to this
  such as rapid heartbeat and
  breathing, insomnia, fatigue
- *digestive*: calms stomach muscles,
  relieves indigestion, upset stomach
  and painful digestion
- *immune*: mild stimulant, which helps
  body recover after illness.

When shouldn't it be used?
Petitgrain has no known ill-effects.

If you remember only one thing...
Petitgrain is a great stress-reliever and
anti-depressant.

Pine (Common/Scotch)

There are many varieties of pine so it is wise to check the botanical name to ensure that you get the right one. Scotch pine is generally safe but Dwarf pine is hazardous and should not be used.

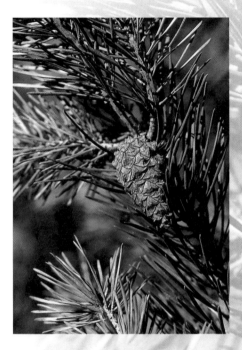

What is its botanical name?
Pinus sylvestris.

Where in the world does it come from?
Pine trees grow all over the world. Trees from northern countries such as Finland, Norway and Russia are said to produce the best oil.

Which part of the plant is used to make the oil?
The pine needles.

How is it extracted?
By distillation of the dry needles.

What is its chemical make-up?
Pine is mostly pinenes (T-erpene). Anything from 50-90% of the oil is terpenes, including pinene, limonene, myrcene, carene and dipentene. Its chemical make-up is T.

What are its therapeutic actions?
Pine is
- antiseptic
- antispasmodic
- bactericidal
- deodorant
- expectorant
- refreshing
- antimicrobial
- vermifuge
- stimulant
- uplifting.

Which conditions/systems benefit from its use?
- *skin*: antiseptic use for congested or infected skins
- *skeletal*: relieves aches and pains in joints, eases rheumatism
- *circulatory*: stimulates circulation
- *nervous*: refreshes and stimulates weak, lethargic, fatigued minds
- *endocrine*: balances male endocrine system
- *respiratory*: clears mucus and acts as antiseptic for flu, colds, bronchitis, coughs, decongests sinuses and nose
- *urinary*: cystitis, urinary tract infections
- *general*: revitalises body, deodorises.

When shouldn't it be used?
For sensitive skin or skin that is allergic or easily irritated.

If you remember only one thing...
Pine is invigorating, refreshing and cleansing: think of how many air fresheners, deodorants and cleaning products (either household or cosmetic) use pine as a fragrance!

Rose (cabbage)

Cabbage rose is sometimes known as French rose. Distilled rose oil is known as rose otto.

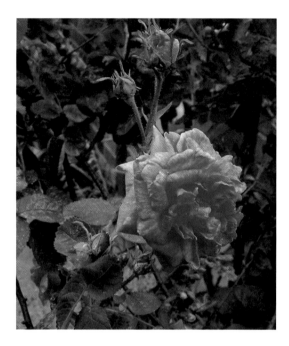

What is its botanical name?
Rosa centifolia.

Where in the world does it come from?
Mediterranean countries like Morocco, France, Italy and Tunisia. It is also grown in China.

Which part of the plant is used to make the oil?
The flower petals.

How is it extracted?
The best oil comes from direct/steam distillation. However, a lot of rose oil is solvent extracted, producing a concrete and then absolute.

What is its chemical make-up?
Cabbage rose is citronellol (18-22%) geraniol and nerol (Al-Cohols), phenyl ethyl alcohol (an aromatic Al-Cohol) plus stearopten (a solid hydrocarbon found in rose oil that has cooled and solidified; a form of T-erpene) and others. Its chemical make-up is AC- T.

What are its therapeutic actions?
Cabbage rose is
- antidepressant
- antiseptic
- antispasmodic
- antiviral
- astringent
- bactericidal
- depurative
- emmenagogue
- haemostatic
- relaxing
- sedative
- laxative
- tonic
- vasoconstrictive.

Which conditions/systems benefit from its use?
- *skin*: vasoconstrictor thus reduces inflammations, broken capillaries and thread veins; dry, mature skin and wrinkles; eczema
- *nervous*: rose oil is a very effective anti-depressant and also helps relieve symptoms of nervous tension and stress as well as insomnia; stimulates positive emotions, thus combating jealousy, sadness, grief; balancing
- *reproductive*: regulates menstrual problems and uterine disorders, calms PMT, increases semen production; relaxing thus helps impotence/ frigidity.

When shouldn't it be used?
Distilled rose oil has no known contra-indications, however, as a precaution it should not be used in pregnancy.

If you remember only one thing...
Cabbage and damask rose have very similar properties but cabbage rose is said to be more aphrodisiac and more relaxing than damask.

Rose (damask)

Damask rose (sometimes known as Bulgarian rose), like jasmine, is one of the best and the most expensive of essential oils. However, it can be used sparingly to great effect so it may be worth the investment. Distilled rose oil is known as rose otto.

What is its botanical name?
Rosa damascena.

Where in the world does it come from?
Rosa damascena is native to Asia but is mostly cultivated in Bulgaria, Turkey and France.

Which part of the plant is used to make the oil?
The flower petals.

How is it extracted?
The best oil comes from water/steam distillation. However, a lot of rose oil is solvent extracted, producing a concrete and then absolute.

What is its chemical make-up?
Rose is mostly citronellol (34-55%), geraniol and nerol (30-40%) (all Al-Cohols), plus 19-22% stearopten (a solid hydrocarbon found in rose oil that has cooled and solidified; a form of T-erpene) and a small amount of phenyl

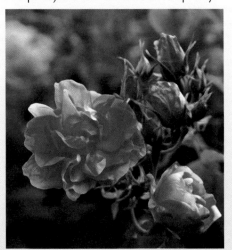

ethyl alcohol (an aromatic Al-Cohol) plus trace elements. Its chemical make-up is AC-T.

What are its therapeutic actions?
Damask rose is
- antidepressant
- antiseptic
- antispasmodic
- antiviral
- astringent
- bactericidal
- depurative
- emmenagogue
- haemostatic
- relaxing
- sedative
- laxative
- tonic
- vasoconstrictive.

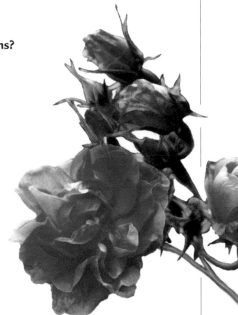

Which conditions/systems benefit from its use?
- *skin*: vasoconstrictor thus reduces inflammations, broken capillaries and thread veins; dry, mature skin and wrinkles; eczema
- *nervous*: rose oil is a very effective antidepressant and also helps relieve symptoms of nervous tension and stress as well as insomnia; stimulates positive emotions, thus combating jealousy, sadness, grief; balancing
- *reproductive*: regulates menstrual problems and uterine disorders, calms PMT, increases semen production; relaxing thus helps impotence/ frigidity.

When shouldn't it be used?
Distilled rose oil has no known contra-indications, however, as a precaution it should not be used in pregnancy.

If you remember only one thing...
Damask rose is especially effective for emotional and reproductive problems. It is also said to be an aphrodisiac...!

Rosemary

Rosemary is from the same plant family as lavender and, like its relative, it has many uses in aromatherapy.

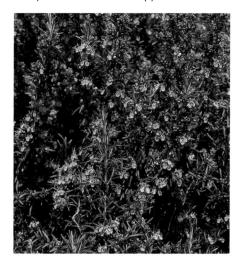

What is its botanical name?
Rosmarinus officinalis.

Where in the world does it come from?
Rosemary grows all over the world but it comes mainly from Mediterranean countries such as France, Spain and Italy.

Which part of the plant is used to make the oil?
The leaves and flowers of the herb.

How is it extracted?
By steam distillation.

What is its chemical make-up?
Rosemary is mostly T-erpenes like pinene, camphene and limonene, plus Al-Cohols (linalol and borneol) and camphor (K-etone). Its chemical make-up is T-AC-K.

What are its therapeutic actions?
Rosemary is
- analgesic
- antiseptic
- antispasmodic
- antiviral
- astringent
- cephalic
- diuretic
- emmenagogue
- hypertensive
- rubefacient
- stimulant
- nervine
- vulnerary
- cordial
- tonic
- uplifting.

Which conditions/systems benefit from its use?
- *skin*: effective astringent, eases puffiness and clears congested dull skin
- *skeletal*: joint problems including arthritis, rheumatism, bursitis
- *muscular*: pain relief for sport/exercise-related injuries/pains
- *circulatory*: rubefacient thus stimulates poor circulation, tonifies heart, improves low blood pressure
- *nervous*: refreshes and clears the mind; improves and aids memory; relieves mental fatigue and lethargy; also activates the brain and stimulates nerve endings (useful for stroke patients); relieves headaches, migraines and vertigo
- *respiratory*: flu, colds, sinusitis, chest infections
- *general*: diuretic thus aids fluid retention and obesity.

When shouldn't it be used?
During pregnancy or for those with epilepsy or high blood pressure.

If you remember only one thing...
Rosemary, like lavender is a good all-round oil, stimulating both mind and body and especially useful for PMT, circulatory problems and infections.

Rosewood

Rosewood is grown in Latin America and the trees form part of the rainforests which are under constant threat at present. Any aromatherapist concerned about the environmental effects of cutting down these forests (which is necessary to obtain the oil) can ease their conscience by looking for rosewood from controlled and cultivated plantations (see Davis, *Aromatherapy: an A-Z*, pp. 263-64.)

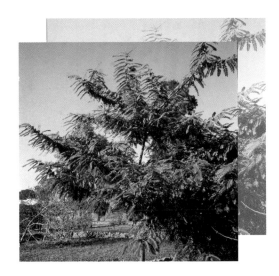

What is its botanical name?
Aniba rosaeodora. *NB Avoid ocotea which is often sold as a substitute.*

Where in the world does it come from?
Brazil, Peru.

Which part of the plant is used to make the oil?
The wood chippings.

How is it extracted?
Steam distillation.

What is its chemical make-up?
Rosewood is mostly Al-cohols (AC), especially linalol, geraniol and terpineol, plus cineol (O-xide). Its chemical make-up is AC-O.

What are its therapeutic actions?
Rosewood is
- analgesic (mild)
- antidepressant
- antiseptic
- antimicrobial
- bactericidal
- cytophylactic
- cephalic
- deodorant
- stimulant
- tonic.

Which conditions/systems benefit from its use?
- *skin*: cell-regenerator thus useful for dry, mature and/or wrinkled skin; also tonic for sensitive skin, acne, dermatitis
- *nervous*: analgesic on headaches, eases stress-related conditions and nervous tension; clears the mind
- *immune*: improves immunity thus effective at protecting against colds, flu and infections
- *general*: deodorises, tonifies.

When shouldn't it be used?
Rosewood has no known contra-indications.

If you remember only one thing...
Rosewood is an extremely effective anti-depressant. It 'lifts' anyone who uses it.

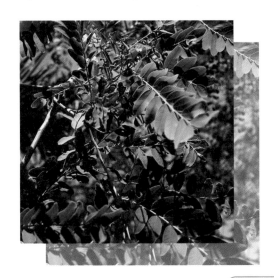

Sandalwood

Sandalwood has been used for medical and therapeutic purposes for over 4000 years.

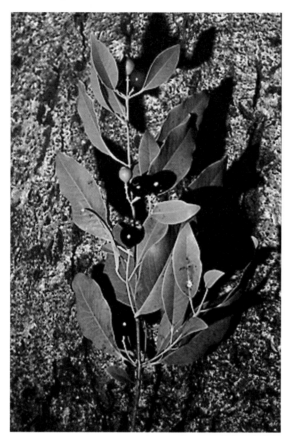

What is its chemical make-up?

Sandalwood is mostly santalol (Al-Cohol) and sesquiterpenes (T-erpene) such as santene and santalene. Its chemical make-up is AC-T.

What are its therapeutic actions?

Sandalwood is

- antidepressant
- antispasmodic
- antiseptic
- bactericidal
- expectorant
- relaxing
- sedative
- tonic.

Which conditions/systems benefit from its use?

- *skin*: soothes dry, irritated, chapped skins; eczema; sensitive skins, calms redness of broken capillaries and reduces high colouring
- *nervous*: soothes tension, relieves stress, insomnia and anxiety
- *respiratory*: throat and chest infections, bronchitis; sedates dry, tickly coughs
- *urinary*: infections, cystitis, cleansing effect on kidneys.

Did you know?

Many male toiletries contain sandalwood.

What is its botanical name?

Santalum album.

Where in the world does it come from?

East India, Sri Lanka and Australia.

Which part of the plant is used to make the oil?

Timber, inner heartwood and roots.

How is it extracted?

Steam distillation.

When shouldn't it be used?

Sandalwood has no known contra-indications.

If you remember only one thing...

Sandalwood is widely used in perfumes and is a relaxing and soothing oil, especially good for calming irritations, whether of the nerves, skin or chest.

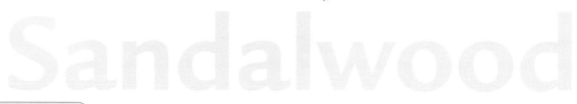

Tea tree
(sometimes spelt Ti tree)

What is its botanical name?
Melaleuca alternifolia.

Where in the world does it come from?
Australia.

Which part of the plant is used to make the oil?
The leaves and twigs of the tree.

How is it extracted?
Steam/direct distillation.

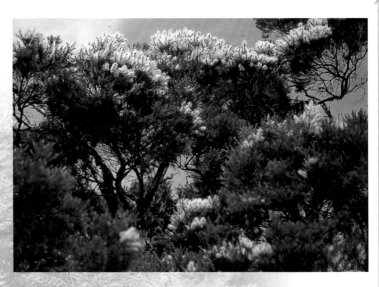

What is its chemical make-up?
Tea tree is mostly terpinene (T-erpene), cineol (O-xide), pinene (T-erpene) plus other S-esquiterpenes. Its chemical make-up is T-O-T-S.

What are its therapeutic actions?
Tea tree is
- anti-inflammatory
- antiseptic
- antiviral
- bactericidal
- cooling
- fungicidal
- immuno-stimulant
- sudorific
- vulnerary
- tonic.

Which conditions/systems benefit from its use?
- *skin*: any fungal or viral infections: cold sores and spots (used neat), acne, athlete's foot, warts, verrucas; infected wounds or boils; blisters, burns, sunburn, dandruff, general itching
- *lymphatic*: glandular fever
- *nervous*: revitalises the mind
- *respiratory*: flu, colds, catarrh, promotes sweating so can reduce fever
- *urinary*: thrush, cystitis, urinary tract infections
- *immune*: boosts the immune system, thus can help shorten time of illness by helping body's defences to fight back
- *general*: useful to prepare body for an operation and to help it recover.

When shouldn't it be used?
Tea tree is generally safe but can irritate the skin in some cases.

If you remember only one thing...
Tea tree is a rarity amongst oils in that it has been proven to have an effect on all three types of infection that attack the body: bacteria, viruses and fungi (see Davis, *Aromatherapy: an A-Z*, p. 295). It is therefore useful both for treating infection and preventing it. It is *the* all-round first-aid oil.

Vetiver

What is its botanical name?
Vetiveria zizanoides.

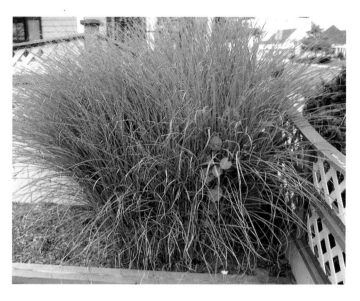

Where in the world does it come from?
It is native to South India and Indonesia but is also cultivated throughout the world, in South America, Reunion, Java and Haiti.

Which part of the plant is used to make the oil?
The underground roots of the grass.

How is it extracted?
By steam distillation.

What is its chemical make-up?
Vetiver is mostly vetiverol (Al-Cohol), vitivone (K-etone) and vetivenes (T-erpenes). Its chemical make-up is AC-K-T.

What are its therapeutic actions?
Vetiver is
- relaxing
- rubefacient
- sedative
- stimulant
- vermifuge
- nervine
- tonic.

Which conditions/systems benefit from its use?
- *skin*: helps heal acne scars
- *muscular*: eases aches and pains
- *circulatory*: increases blood flow, strengthens red blood cells, calms palpitations
- *nervous*: the mind benefits the most from vetiver; it calms the central nervous system, reduces tension, worry, anxiety and any stress-related symptoms; relieves insomnia and nervous debility
- *reproductive*: tonic.

When shouldn't it be used?
Vetiver has no known contraindications.

If you remember only one thing...
Vetiver is the oil of tranquillity. It has a tranquillising, grounding effect, bringing the user back down to earth, helping relaxation and the release of mental and physical exhaustion.

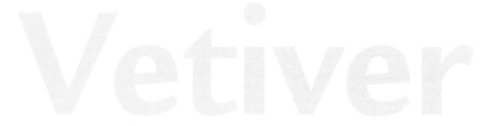

Ylang ylang

What is its botanical name?
Cananga odorata.

Where in the world does it come from?
Indonesia, the Philippines, Madagascar.

Which part of the plant is used to make the oil?
Flower petals.

How is it extracted?
By steam distillation.

What is its chemical make-up?
Ylang ylang is mostly methyl benzoate, methyl salicylate and benzyl acetate (all E-sters), linalol and geraniol (Al-Cohols), plus some T-erpenes such as pinene. Its chemical make-up is E-AC-T.

What are its therapeutic actions?
Ylang ylang is
- antidepressant
- aphrodisiac
- hypotensive
- relaxing
- sedative
- tonic.

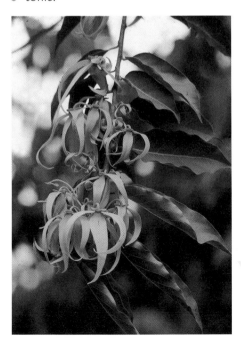

Which conditions/systems benefit from its use?
- *skin*: balances sebum production both for oily and dry skins; extractive effect on acne i.e. draws out the spot and infection (so it will get worse before getting better)
- *circulatory*: slows over-rapid breathing (hyperpnoea) and heartbeat (tachycardia); reduces high blood pressure
- *nervous*: antidepressant, creates feelings of joy, calms central nervous system
- *endocrine*: regulates flow of adrenaline and thus slows its effects reducing stress, anger, frustration, panic, fear and shock; balances hormones
- *reproductive*: tonic for womb; impotence, frigidity.

When shouldn't it be used?
Ylang ylang has a very heady perfume and can cause headaches and nausea. It should therefore be used in moderation.

If you remember only one thing...
Ylang ylang has a euphoric effect, promoting positive emotions in the user and calming and sedating in times of stress.

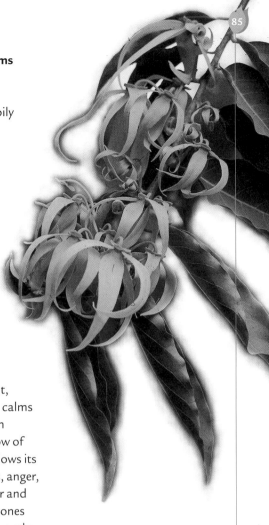

Ylang ylang

Where in the world? This map shows the country of origin of some essential oils.

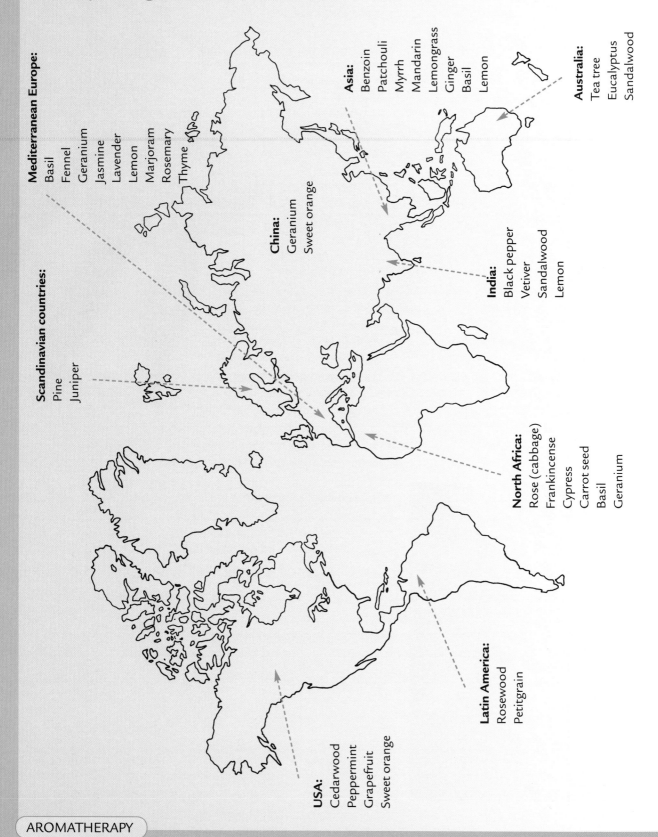

Scandinavian countries:
Pine
Juniper

Mediterranean Europe:
Basil
Fennel
Geranium
Jasmine
Lavender
Lemon
Marjoram
Rosemary
Thyme

China:
Geranium
Sweet orange

Asia:
Benzoin
Patchouli
Myrrh
Mandarin
Lemongrass
Ginger
Basil
Lemon

Australia:
Tea tree
Eucalyptus
Sandalwood

India:
Black pepper
Vetiver
Sandalwood
Lemon

North Africa:
Rose (cabbage)
Frankincense
Cypress
Carrot seed
Basil
Geranium

USA:
Cedarwood
Peppermint
Grapefruit
Sweet orange

Latin America:
Rosewood
Petitgrain

A–Z Revision Table

Name	Part of plant	Country	Main constituents	Extraction method	Safety factors	Aroma use
Basil (*Ocimum basilicum*)	Flowering herb	Asia & Africa Now Europe	Linalol Eugenol	Steam distillation	Avoid during pregnancy	Antiseptic Antispasmodic Headaches Uplifting/refreshing Digestion
Benzoin (*Styrax benzoin*)	Directly from the trees – resin	Tropical Asia	Coniferyl Cinnamate Sumaresinolic acid	Solvent extraction	Possible skin sensitisation	Inflamed skin Good for stress Warming/relaxing Respiratory Circulation
Bergamot (*Citrus bergamia*)	Fruit (Similar to an orange)	Tropical Asia Southern Italy (cultivated)	Linalyl Acetate Linalol	Cold expression from peel	Can be phototoxic (if contains Bergapten which is a furocoumarin: a phototoxic ingredient)	Anxiety Depression Nervous system Immune system Uplifting Cooling
Black pepper (*Piper nigrum*)	Fruit	Native to South-west India. Major producers are India, Indonesia, Malaysia, China	Pinene Camphene	Steam distillation from black peppercorns dried and crushed	Irritant – use in moderation. Not compatible with homeopathic treatments	Muscular aches and pains Circulatory problems Stimulating Coughs and colds
Carrot seed (*Daucus carota*)	Seed	Europe Asia N.Africa	Carotol Daucol	Steam distillation of seeds	Avoid during pregnancy	Mature skins Rejuvenating Stress-related skin diseases PMT Liver congestion
Chamomile (German) (blue) (*Matricaria recutica* or *Matricaria chamomilla*)	Flower	Europe. Cultivated extensively in Hungary and Eastern Europe	Chamazulene – produced during distillation Farnesol	Steam distillation	Causes dermatitis in some people	Allergies Inflammation Skin conditions (calms) Bruising Insomnia Stress Relaxing
Chamomile (Roman) (*Chamaemelum nobile* or *anthemis*)	Flower	Europe and the USA	Angelic/tiglic acids	Steam distillation	Causes dermatitis in some people	Same as German but stronger

Name	Part used	Origin	Constituents	Extraction	Cautions	Properties / Uses
Clary Sage (*Salvia sclarea*)	Flowering tops or tops and seed	Russia and Southern Europe	Linalylacetate Linalol	Steam distillation	Narcotic: alcohol should not be drunk when using it. Avoid during pregnancy	Nervous tension Panic Joints Muscles Muscles Relaxing
Coriander (*Coriandrum sativum*)	Seeds	Russia Europe Western Asia	Linalol Borneol	Steam distillation	Use in moderation	Arthritis Muscular aches and pains Nausea Immune system Nervous exhaustion
Cypress (*Cupressus sempervirens*)	Cones Twigs	Eastern Mediterranean	Pinene Camphene	Steam distillation	Avoid during pregnancy	Excessive perspiration Cellulite Oedema Poor circulation Lymph Haemorrhoids & varicose veins
Eucalyptus (*Eucalyptus globulus*)	Leaves and twigs	Tasmania and Australia Coastal Mediterranean – Spain	Cineol Limonene	Steam distillation	Not compatible with homeopathic treatments	Headaches Head clearing Immune Respiratory Sinusitis Stimulating
Fennel (sweet) (*Foeniculum vulgare* var. *dulce*)	Crushed seeds	Cultivated extensively in France, Italy and Greece	Limonene Anethole	Steam distillation	Non-irritant Non-toxic Narcotic in large doses Do not use in pregnancy or if epileptic Never use bitter fennel on the skin	Dull complexions Cellulite Oedema Constipation Amenorrhea Menopause Carminative (eases stomach pains/wind) Digestion
Frankincense (*Boswellia carteri*)	From the gum resin which is collected by making incisions into the bark	Native to the Red Sea region. Grows wild throughout North-east Africa	Pinene Limonene	Steam distillation	None known	Mature skins Asthma and bronchitis Anxiety and nervous tension Immune system Sedative Meditation
Geranium (*Pelargonium graveolens*)	Leaves, stalks and flowers	Native to South Africa. Three main regions for essential oil production: Mediterranean Europe, Egypt and Russia	Geraniol Citronellol	Steam distillation	Non-toxic Non-irritant Non-sensitising Possible dermatitis in hypersensitive individuals	Very good for circulatory problems and oedema Endocrine: PMT, menopause, helps adrenal glands Nervous tension and stress-related conditions

	Part used	Origin	Main constituents	Extraction	Cautions	Properties/Uses
(Zingiber officinale)			...acid	May cause sensitisation	Digestive	
Grapefruit (*Citrus paradisi*)	Fresh peel	Tropical Asia & West Indies	Limonene Cadinene	Expression	Non-toxic	Circulation Oedema/cellulite Depression Nervous exhaustion Refreshing Uplifting
Jasmine (*Jasmine officinale*)	Flowers	China, Northern India, Eygpt and France	Benzyl Acetate Linalol	Solvent extraction which produces an absolute. This is steam distilled	Non toxic May cause an allergic reaction	Nervous instability, depression Hydrates Labour pains
Juniper (*Juniperus communis*)	1 Berry 2 Twigs and needles	Scandinavia Siberia Canada	Pinene Myrcene	Steam distillation	Nephrotoxic-irritates kidneys. Never use with history of kidney conditions Never use during pregnancy	Nervous exhaustion Stress-related conditions Circulation De-toxifying Cellulite
Lavender (*Lavandula angustifolia*)	Flowering tops, leaves, stems	Mediterranean	Linalyl acetate Lavandulyl acetate	Steam distillation	None known	Very versatile Antibacterial and germicidal Skincare/burns, wounds Good for stress relief, relaxation, insomnia Circulation Immune system Nervous system Refreshing and relaxing
Lemon (*Citrus limon*)	Outer part of the fresh peel	Native to Asia, probably East India	Limonene Pinene	Cold expression from outer part of fresh peel	May cause skin sensitisation or irritation; phototoxic	Acne Circulatory problems Lowers blood pressure Arthritis Rheumatism Colds, flu, etc Immune system Refreshing Stimulating
Lemongrass (*Cymbopogon citratus*)	Fresh and partially dried leaves (grass) finely chopped	West Indies East India	Citral Geraniol	Steam distillation	Possible dermal irritation – use with care	Antiseptic Nervous exhaustion Stress-related conditions Circulation Muscles & joints
Lime (*Citrus medica*)	Peel, whole fruit	Asia Europe West Indies Americas	Limonene Pinene	Expression/ Steam distillation	Phototoxic when expressed	Acne and oily skins Cellulite Fatigue Colds and flu Immune system

Oil	Part used	Origin	Constituents	Extraction	Cautions	Properties and uses
Mandarin (Citrus reticulata)	Outer peel	Native to China and Far East	Limonene, Methyl anthranilate	Essential oil by cold expression	Possibly phototoxic	Anxiety; Insomnia; Stomach ailments; Uplifting; Refreshing; Stretch marks; Oedema; Digestive
Marjoram (sweet) (Origanum marjorana)	Dried flowering herb and leaves	Native to Mediterranean region, Egypt and North Africa	Terpineol, Linalol	Essential oil by steam distillation	Avoid during pregnancy	Muscular aches and pains; Headaches; Circulation; Relaxant; Helps insomnia; Stress
Melissa (Lemon balm) (Melissa officinalis)	Leaves and flowers. Very often several oils are blended to simulate melissa because it is so expensive to obtain	Mediterranean region	Citral, Geraniol	Steam distillation	May cause skin irritation but should be used well diluted	Most types of stress relief; Shock; Ideal for PMT; Relaxing; High blood pressure
Myrrh (Commiphora myrrha)	Oleo gum Resin incised tree bark Crude myrrh	Red Sea Area Ethiopia Sudan N.E Africa	Heerabolene, Limonene	Resinoid by solvent extraction Essential oil by steam distillation	Not to be used during pregnancy Toxic in high quantities	Anti-inflammatory; Mature skin; Fungal infections; Athlete's foot; Respiratory problems; Colds and flu; Cooling and toning
Neroli (Orange blossom) (Citrus aurantium var. amara)	Orange blossom flowers	Italy, France, North Africa, native to Far East	Linalol, Limonene	Concrete and absolute can be produced by solvent extraction; essential oil by steam distillation	None known	Stress relief; Anxiety; Insomnia; Nervous system; Eases palpitations; Mature skins; Emotional upsets; Very relaxing
Niaouli (Melaleuca viridiflora)	Leaves and twigs	Australia Tasmania	Cineole, Terpineol	Steam distillation	Often subject to adulteration	Insect bites; Rheumatism; Muscular aches and pains; Urinary infections; Coughs and sore throats; Cystitis
Orange (sweet) (Citrus sinensis)	Outer peel	Mediterranean	Limonene, Bergapten	Cold expression or steam distillation	If distilled is phototoxic	Dull oily skin; Digestion; Nervous tension; Stress-related conditions; Refreshing

Oil	Part used	Origin	Constituents	Extraction	Cautions	Uses
Palmarosa (*Cymbopogon martinii*)	Fresh/dried grass	India, Comoro Islands, Africa, Indonesia	Geraniol, Farnesol	Steam distillation	None	Skin infections, Acne, Digestive problems, Nervous exhaustion, Stress-related conditions
Patchouli (*Pogostemon cablin*)	Dried leaves	Indonesia, Philippines	Patchouli alcohol, Patchoulol	Steam distillation	May cause photo-toxicity. Use in low concentrations	Insect repellent, Nervous conditions, Scarred tissue
Peppermint (*Mentha piperita*)	Flowers and leaves	Worldwide	Menthol, Menthones	Steam distillation	Not compatible with homeopathy; possible sensitisation so use well-diluted	Indigestion, Flatulence, Headaches, Cooling/refreshing, Cephalic, Nervous system, Immune system
Petitgrain (*Citrus aurantium* var. *amara*)	Leaves and twigs of bitter orange	Mediterranean	Linalyl acetate, Geranyl acetate	Steam distillation	None known	Insomnia, Nervous exhaustion, Stress-related conditions, Relieves indigestion
Pine (Common/Scotch) (*Pinus sylvestris*)	Needles	Finland, Norway, Russia	Pinenes, Limonene	Dry distillation of the needles	May cause skin irritation if used at high levels. Avoid in allergic skin conditions	Respiratory, Circulatory, Immune system, Urinary infections
Rose (cabbage) (*Rosa centifolia*)	Flowers	Mediterranean	Citronellol, Geraniol	Steam distillation	Avoid during pregnancy	Dry skin, Eczema, Mature/sensitive skin, Uterine disorders, Impotence, Irregular menstruation, Frigidty, PMT, Depression
Rose (damask) (*Rosa damascena*)	Petals	Bulgaria, Turkey, France	Citronellol, Geraniol	Steam distillation	Avoid during pregnancy	As above.
Rosemary (*Rosmarinus officinalis*)	Leaves and flowers	Native to Mediterranean	Camphene, Pinenes	Steam distillation	Avoid during pregnancy. Do not use on epileptics. Contraindicated in cases of high blood pressure	Stimulates mind, Congested skin, Muscle/joint aches, Headaches, Immune system, Stress-related disorders, Invigorating, Refreshing

Name	Part used	Origin	Constituents	Extraction	Cautions	Uses
Rosewood (Anaeba rosaeodora)	Wood chippings	Brazil / Peru	Linalol / Geraniol	Steam distillation	None known	Skin conditions / Mature skin / Sensitive / Immune system / Stress
Sandalwood (Santalum album)	Wood	Native to tropical Asia	Santalol / Santene	Steam distillation	None known	Skin ailments / Throat and chest infections / Dry/sensitive skin / Stress / Depression / Insomnia / Powerful antiseptic / Relaxing/calming
Tea tree (Melaleuca alternifolia)	Leaves and twigs	Australia	Terpinene / Cineol	Steam/water distillation	Possible skin sensitisation	Any infections / Coughs and colds / Thrush / Cystitis / Antiseptic / Antibacterial / First-aid kit in a bottle / Anxiety / Warming
Vetiver (Vetiveria zizanoides)	Roots of the grass	South India / Indonesia / Sri Lanka	Vetiverol / Vitivone	Steam distillation	None known	Nervous system / Deeply relaxing / Calming / Good for stress / Palpitations / Hyperactivity / Anxiety / Hyperventilation
Ylang Ylang (Cananga odorata)	Freshly picked flowers	Tropical Asia / Philippines / Indonesia	Methyl benzoate / Methyl salicylate	Steam distillation. First extraction is Ylang Ylang which is top grade, plus three further distillates	Use in moderation / Can cause headaches or nausea	Stress reduction / Hyperventilation / Anxiety / Mental relaxant / Calming / Antidepressant / Relaxing / Aphrodisiac / High blood pressure / Palpitations

6 How to use essential oils at home

Putting drops of essential oil into a burner.

In Brief

This chapter explains the different and most effective methods of using essential oils at home.

Essential oils are very easy to use at home for medical and non-medical purposes. Many common ailments can be treated by using oils in the bath, in creams and lotions and in steam inhalations.

NB a medical professional and/or professional aromatherapist should be consulted for serious medical and psychological conditions.

Massage

Massage is the most common application method. The warmth of the hands helps to move the oil across the skin and work it into the affected area. The essential oil should be blended with the chosen carrier oil (see Chapter 4 for more detailed information on blending and carrier oils) in the following dilutions:

1. 2 drops to 5ml (one teaspoon) for adults
2. 6 drops to 15ml (three teaspoons or one tablespoon)
3. 20 drops to 50ml (10 teaspoons).

Once blended, essential oils will share the shelf life of the carrier oil they are mixed with so it is best not to mix more than is needed. The following suggested amounts will obviously need to be adapted for smaller/larger frames, children and the elderly:

1. a face massage requires 5ml carrier oil
2. a full body massage requires 20-25ml carrier oil
3. a specific area of the body (e.g. hands, feet, arm, neck) may require from 5-15ml oil.

Compresses

A compress is a piece of material that has been soaked in water and is then placed over an affected part of the body and held in place for a period of time. Both hot and cold compresses can be used: hot compresses are more useful for muscular aches and pains, earaches and toothaches whereas cold compresses are

better for joint sprains and headaches. Essential oil is mixed with the water before adding the material. To make a compress:

1. fill a bowl with 100mls of hot or cold water and add one drop of the chosen essential oil
2. soak a piece of material (e.g. a flannel or unmedicated gauze) in the bowl of water
3. squeeze out the excess water and place the material over the affected area
4. cover with cling film to hold the material in place and leave for approximately two hours
5. the compress will soon cool down/warm up. Repeat the process as long as is necessary/desired.

Baths

Probably the easiest and most everyday way to use essential oils is to put them in the bath. Remember, though, that essential oils do not dissolve in water and will only float or sink. Therefore they should be mixed with a small quantity of

A foot bath.

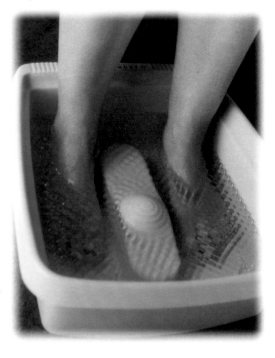

an emulsifier, preferably unperfumed, such as shampoo, liquid soap, shower gel, or even full cream milk before adding them to the bath. Skin irritants (e.g. spicy oils such as black pepper) are not recommended for a relaxing bath! To use oils in the bath:

- run a hot, but not over-hot, bath
- close the doors and windows (this seals the aromatic scent in the room for maximum benefit)
- mix up to six drops of essential oil in a carrier oil, or emulsifier such as milk or fragrance-free shampoo/shower gel/bath foam
- add the mixture to the water soak and enjoy!

Baths can also be used for a particular part of the body. For a foot/hand bath mix two drops of essential oil in a bowl of warm water and soak the affected foot/hand for about 20 minutes. For haemorrhoids, childbirth stitches and genital infections like thrush, sitting in a warm bath (known as a sitz bath) containing two or three drops of essential oil can help. Again the oils should be mixed with an emulsifier. Tea tree is good for thrush and lavender oil helps healing after childbirth.

Vaporisers

Essential oils can be vaporised (warmed so that they evaporate and spread their aroma around a room) either in an oil burner, on a light bulb ring or using the heat of a radiator.

- **Burner**: burners are usually a small bowl placed over a nightlight candle. The heat from the candle evaporates whatever is in the bowl. It is best to use a glazed, non-porous burner. Put water in the small bowl, add two drops of the chosen essential oil to the water and light the candle. The bowl should not be allowed to burn dry because this causes a bitter smell. Burners can be used for general

atmosphere (e.g. to relax, uplift, soothe) or for more specific purposes such as keeping insects away (lemongrass is a good insect repellent).

- **Light bulbs**: the heat from a light bulb can be used to evaporate essential oils. About two drops of oil is usually enough for each use. Light bulb rings and attachments should be fitted when the light is off and the bulb is cool.
- **Radiators**: place two drops of essential oil onto a cotton wool ball and place it on, or behind a radiator when it is on. The heat from the radiator will evaporate the oil.

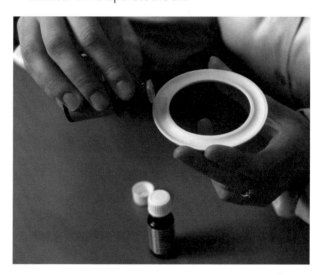

Putting drops of essential oil onto a light bulb ring.

Inhalation

Essential oils can be added to very hot water and then inhaled in the steam. This is very effective for respiratory problems and sinus infections, clearing the mucus and blocked noses associated with colds and flu. It is also good for brightening the complexion and clearing the skin of blocked pores and excess oil. Steam inhalation is not recommended for asthmatics.

1. fill a bowl, or a sink, with hot water
2. add two drops of the chosen essential oil (eucalyptus and peppermint are good for respiratory infections; tea tree helps the skin)

3. lean over the bowl, not too close to the water, and cover your head with a cloth or towel so that the bowl is enclosed by the material (which helps keep the oil's valuable aroma close to the affected area)
4. keeping eyes closed, inhale the steam for several minutes.

Creams, lotions and face masks

Many commercially-produced face creams, masks and body lotions contain essential oils but it is easy and cheaper to make your own. Any unperfumed cream or lotion can be mixed with a few drops of essential oil to make an individually perfumed product. It is best to use a home-made cream or one which clearly states its contents, since some may contain chemicals that react with the essential oil, or counteract its therapeutic effects. Some of the most suitable creams are sold by suppliers of essential oils. Follow the dilutions used for massage oils (i.e. two drops of essential oil per 5ml teaspoon of cream/lotion). A basic face mask, either home-made or commercial, can be customised with a drop of essential oil. To prevent skin reactions, oils known to cause irritation should be avoided.

Flower waters (hydrolats)

Steam distillation of a plant to extract the essential oil produces an oily water (see Chapter 2 for more details). The essential oil floats to the top and is separated off, leaving water which will be scented by traces of the oil (for example distillation of lavender will produce lavender oil and lavender water). This is a hydrolat or flower water. Hydrolats do not contain essential oils but they do take up some of the fragrance. They are safe to use neat without further dilution unless labelled otherwise. Hydrolats have similar therapeutic qualities to the oil they derive from, even though they are not as pure and do not have exactly the same chemical make-up: thus just as lavender oil is versatile so is lavender water. They have been used for centuries in skin preparations and perfumes. Flower waters can be used for cosmetic purposes (rose water and orange-flower water are both sold as skin tonics) or for the treatment of skin conditions, especially those like eczema which would be aggravated by using a cream. They can also be used around the house, e.g. in baths or for scenting pot pourri. In the Mediterranean and North Africa, orange-flower water is used in cooking, for scenting cakes and dishes such as couscous. They are very gentle and safe and thus provide a useful introduction to essential oils.

Shampoos

If you have fair hair you may have used a chamomile shampoo in the past, whereas if you have dark hair you may have used a rosemary shampoo (both are said to enhance the different colours). Make your own by mixing two drops of the chosen essential oil with an unperfumed, mild shampoo. Citrus oils will have a refreshing effect on mind and body as will peppermint; flower oils can be used as perfume and soothing oils (like frankincense) will help relaxation.

Neat

Neat application of essential oils, without blending them first or adding them to water, is not recommended. However there are two exceptions. Tea tree can be used neat on spots and lavender oil can be used on wounds and burns.

You now know all the methods of using essential oils at home for common ailments and general well-being. For more serious conditions and problems, a professional aromatherapist should always be consulted.

7 Aromatherapy massage

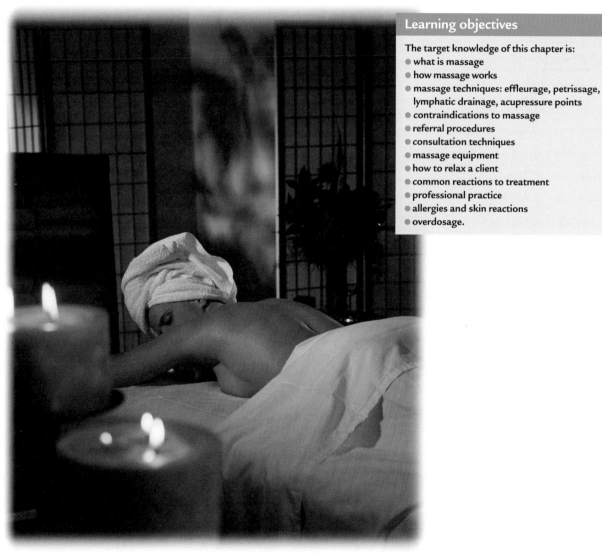

Learning objectives

The target knowledge of this chapter is:
- what is massage
- how massage works
- massage techniques: effleurage, petrissage, lymphatic drainage, acupressure points
- contraindications to massage
- referral procedures
- consultation techniques
- massage equipment
- how to relax a client
- common reactions to treatment
- professional practice
- allergies and skin reactions
- overdosage.

In Brief

This chapter focuses on one particular method of using essential oils, massage. Professionally, this is the most common method of application because the skin absorbs essential oils very easily and effectively. The next chapter explains different massage techniques and how to use them on different parts of the body, as well as explaining certain complementary massage therapies such as acupressure and lymphatic drainage.

WHAT IS MASSAGE?

Massage is the use of the hands to manipulate the soft tissues of the body thus relaxing either a specific area or the whole person. In a way, it is an extension of the basic rub that we give either ourselves, a friend, or a child when we or they bang or knock themselves unexpectedly. Touch is both physically and mentally soothing. It

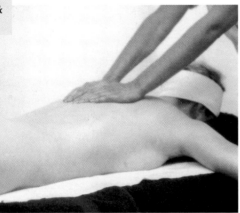

can also be stimulating: think of rubbing the eyes or the face when tired to wake ourselves up, or rubbing an arm or leg that has 'gone to sleep'. All of these actions are forms of massage.

What is aromatherapy massage?

Aromatherapy massage is concerned with relaxing clients and helping them, through the physical and aromatic effects of essential oils, with certain physical and emotional conditions. Using a blend of carrier and essential oils in the correct dilutions, the aromatherapist massages the affected area or the whole body depending on the symptoms and treatment.

You now know what aromatherapy massage is. The next section explains how it works and the different techniques involved.

HOW DOES AROMATHERAPY MASSAGE WORK?

The heat of the hands helps the absorption of the oil by the skin. Different massage techniques encourage relaxation, better circulation, improved suppleness and/or the release of muscular tension.

What are these techniques?

In aromatherapy massage there are two main techniques used: effleurage and petrissage. Both derive from French: effleurer means to touch lightly or to brush against whereas petrissage means to knead or rub with force, like a baker kneading dough. Thus effleurage is a light, soothing stroke whereas petrissage is a more forceful, thorough kneading movement. Lymphatic drainage massage and acupressure are also recommended.

● Effleurage

An effleurage stroke is smooth, gentle and flowing. Pressure is applied slowly, without jerks or breaks, towards the heart (i.e. from the waist towards the shoulders or from the foot towards the thigh). The rhythmic movement helps to relax the client and encourage the release of tension. Effleurage is usually the stroke used to start and finish a massage on a particular limb or area. It can be used in up and down movements or circles. It is a relaxing stroke.

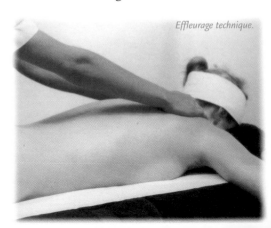

Effleurage technique.

● Petrissage

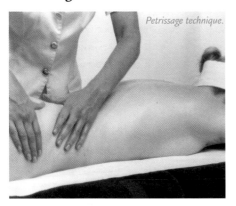

Petrissage technique.

Petrissage is a compression movement and it is therefore only possible on areas of the body where there is enough tissue to compress.

● Lymphatic drainage massage

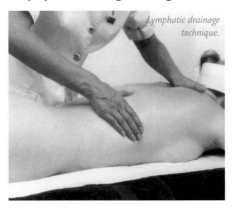

Lymphatic drainage technique.

The lymphatic system is a secondary circulation that aids the removal of waste. It collects toxins and excess fluid from cells and tissues, filters off bacteria, produces antibodies and returns the filtered fluid and antibodies to the blood. Some massage techniques can help the action of the lymphatic system, aiding the removal of toxins and boosting the immune system. It is useful for treating fluid retention or oedema (swelling). Lymphatic drainage massage consists of:

● soft, pumping movements pushing in the direction of the lymph nodes
● light pressure: the lymph vessels are near the surface of the skin so pressure should be gentle not firm.

● Acupressure

Acupressure technique.

Acupressure is a variation of acupuncture, a Chinese therapy. Whereas acupuncture involves inserting very fine needles into certain points in the skin in order to help energy, known as chi, flow more smoothly through the body, acupressure uses finger or thumb pressure on the same points. It can be used during aromatherapy massage to help treat various conditions (see Chapter 9: Other complementary therapies).

Why are continuous movements necessary?

One hand or both should always be kept on the body being massaged during the treatment since as soon as the hands are removed the body will register this as the end of the massage and begin to 'change gear', getting ready to dress and leave.

When is massage not recommended?

Although massage is generally safe it is not advised for use at the following times and for the following clients/conditions:

● pregnancy
● on those receiving medical treatment for a condition
● on those taking drugs/medication (seek advice from a doctor)
● on those recovering from an operation/fracture
● on those recently vaccinated
● serious heart conditions
● infectious or contagious diseases
● fevers/high temperatures
● straight after eating, or after drinking alcohol
● at the start of menstruation
● on broken skin, cuts, wounds
● on varicose veins
● on bruising.

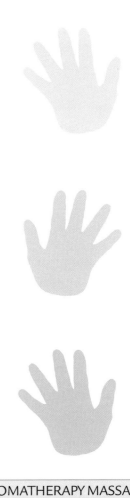

AROMATHERAPY MASSAGE

Seek advice from a doctor/medical practitioner before treating a client with the following:

- angina
- pacemaker
- high/low blood pressure
- thrombosis
- acute rheumatism and arthritis
- slipped discs, torn ligaments or muscles
- epileptics, the paralysed
- Bell's palsy, trapped or pinched nerves
- acute asthma/bronchitis
- kidney infections
- gynaecological infections
- cancer.

Referral procedures

There will be occasions when you are unsure whether to proceed with a treatment. These instances include both the above list and also any other medical conditions, system defects, skin problems or contraindications to medication about which you are uncertain. The best way to approach this is to refer the client to their GP so that they can check whether aromatherapy massage is advisable. It is not the job of the masseur/se to diagnose medical problems or decide if a condition is treatable – in fact the code of conduct of many professional associations, such as the IGPP, states that diagnosis is not allowed); if in doubt, refer the client.

You now know how to use massage and when not to use it. The next section describes the different practicalities required in giving an aromatherapy massage.

CONSULTATION TECHNIQUES

NB For the purpose of this section the person receiving the massage will be known as the client.

Consultation techniques

Before beginning an aromatherapy massage, or a series of massages, the aromatherapist will need to talk to the client in order to find out why they have come for a massage e.g. is it for a medical condition, for a psychological problem (e.g. anxiety, depression) or simply for relaxation? In order to discuss this, clients will need to feel relaxed and, since relaxation is also an important part of the whole massage, the consultation can be a useful way to help both aromatherapist and client to feel comfortable with each other. It also gives the aromatherapist a chance to:
- find out what the client expects
- explain the treatment and the possible effects (i.e. dispelling any unrealistic

or even cynical expectations)
- find out if there are any contra-indications
- select oils that will suit the client and the treatment
- fill out the consultation forms.

The following topics should be covered by a consultation:
- personal details: name, address, telephone number, date of birth, GP's name and address
- medical background: medicines being taken (particularly homeopathic ones which may be incompatible with aromatherapy); medical conditions (any contraindications or problems should be referred; whatever the background a disclaimer form should be sent to the GP for confirmation that aromatherapy will not have any adverse effects); previous illnesses or

hereditary diseases; operations; allergies.

- diet and other factors: eating habits, fluid and alcohol consumption, smoker or non-smoker, sleep problems (like insomnia).

How to carry out a consultation

First, you need a space to consult in. A private, comfortable area, where there will be no interruptions would be suitable. Try to arrange the room/space in an open, inviting way and ensure that your own body language is positive and open e.g. sitting with arms and legs crossed facing away from the client is a very closed and unfriendly stance. Also, sitting behind a desk or standing whilst the client sits may be perceived as threatening. Try to sit facing the client, at the same height, not behind a table or desk. The client must feel relaxed enough to explain the problem/reason that has made them come for an aromatherapy massage. This is where the aromatherapist needs to demonstrate listening and encouraging skills.

How to find out what you need to know

Many clients consulting with an aromatherapist for the first time may be nervous and unwilling to reveal much information about why they have come, either through embarrassment, anxiety or shyness. An open and relaxed person will usually volunteer the required information but with more reticent clients the aromatherapist needs to know how to ask a question as well as how to listen to the answers.

- Start with general questions or, if you want a prompt or sense a particularly shy client, use the form/record card as a starting point. Once you have begun asking questions which are easy to answer (name, address, date of birth etc) the more difficult ones about treatment and contraindications won't seem so daunting – the client will be in the rhythm of responding to your questions and will expect them rather than be made more nervous by them.

- Ask open not closed questions: ones that cannot be answered with yes or no. For example, ask what do you expect from an aromatherapy massage rather than do you expect the massage to work or tell me about your diet rather than do you eat healthily? No one likes to examine their own habits so it is best to address the questions in as open and unthreatening a manner as possible.

- In order to instil trust, use your own body language to encourage and aid

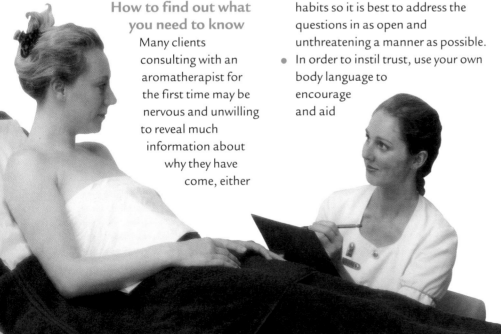

Consulting with a client.

responses: nodding, smiling and leaning forward all communicate interest as does keeping eye contact. Looking away frequently, fidgeting or staring blankly will merely communicate nervousness and/or lack of interest which will not help the client to feel confident in your abilities or your interest in them. Remember that, as an aromatherapist, you are there to help the client: if you are unfriendly, nervous or uncommunicative the client is likely to pick up on this and react in a similar way.

- Be confident, enthusiastic and professional.
- Communicate your own belief and trust in the treatment: this will help the client to believe in it and will improve the psychological and physiological effects of the massage.
- Reassure the client that everything discussed will remain completely confidential and make sure that you never break this confidence.
- Treat everyone equally: if you cannot avoid bringing racist or sexist prejudices to the massage table aromatherapy is not the profession for you.
- Discuss the possible essential oils with the client as fully as is necessary (i.e. describing the effects and qualities of the oils not the chemistry!). The client should smell a couple of oils before you make the final selection. The aroma of the oils, absorbed via the olfactory tract, is vital to the effectiveness of the treatment. Also if there are any selected oils which are unsuitable (due to association or because the client doesn't like the smell) this can be sorted out before the massage begins. It is no good using a blend with geranium on the client if the smell makes him/her feel sick because the oils will not produce the appropriate therapeutic effect.

You now know how to find out the necessary information required to give an effective and safe massage. The next section explains the equipment that is needed and other practical considerations.

WHERE TO GIVE A MASSAGE

Massage requires the person receiving the massage to be partly or completely undressed (underwear should be kept on). The room where the massage takes place should therefore be private and without risk of interruption. Fear of interruption will usually counteract all the positive, relaxing benefits of the massage. It should also be the correct temperature i.e. not too cold or too warm. You will be much warmer than the client because you will be exerting yourself physically. Make sure that there is a suitable ambient temperature. Towels and blankets or heated blankets can help with both these issues. Towels should be placed under and over the client, covering up any area of the body which is not currently being massaged. A blanket may be used on top of the towel at the beginning of the massage or during it, as necessary, to keep the client warm.

What equipment is needed?
- **a massage couch**

In order to comfortably and effectively perform a massage a proper adjustable massage couch is recommended covered with possibly a blanket and then towels. Remember that whoever gives the massage should be comfortable and not adopting bad postures that may cause back or neck ache. A couch that can be adjusted to the right height for each individual prevents such problems.

- **pillows and towels for support and protection**

Pillows will help both client and masseur/se. For a massage of the back, a pillow or face ring under the face/ shoulders and another pillow or supports under the ankles will help improve comfort. Of course, it is best to check with each individual what suits them. For a front of the body massage a pillow under the neck and under the knees will stop them from being unnecessarily stretched and strained during the massage. As mentioned earlier, towels are required to cover the parts of the client which are not being massaged.

- **changing facilities and bathroom**

In a professional situation the client should be able to change and dress in privacy so adequate changing facilities will be required. Also, it is advisable that both masseur/se and client go to the toilet before the massage begins to prevent interruption.

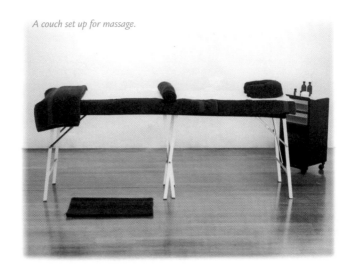

A couch set up for massage.

What about the masseur/se?

The person giving the massage should be dressed comfortably in professional clothes and comfortable shoes. Nails should be kept short, clean and unvarnished and jewellery avoided. Where necessary, hair should be pinned or tied away from the face and collar.

You now know how to set up an area for giving a massage and what equipment is required. The next section explains more intangible considerations: relaxation techniques and good professional practice.

RELAXATION TECHNIQUES AND GOOD PRACTICE

In order for the client to feel relaxed, certain aspects need to be considered. As discussed earlier, the room should be a comfortable temperature, the client's privacy should never be compromised and the masseur/se should be dressed professionally and tidily. Lighting should be bright enough for the massage to be carried out but not harsh: fluorescent and neon lights can often be over-bright. When settling the client on the couch, check that they are comfortable. Some clients may wish to listen to music or talk, some may prefer silence. Remember that

this is their time and you should respect their wishes – they are not paying to hear your views or personal preferences.

Good professional practice

It is extremely important for any aromatherapist to take the following information into consideration when performing a massage.

- **emotions and sex**

When carrying out an aromatherapy massage it is evident that the client will be semi-naked. His or her modesty is of

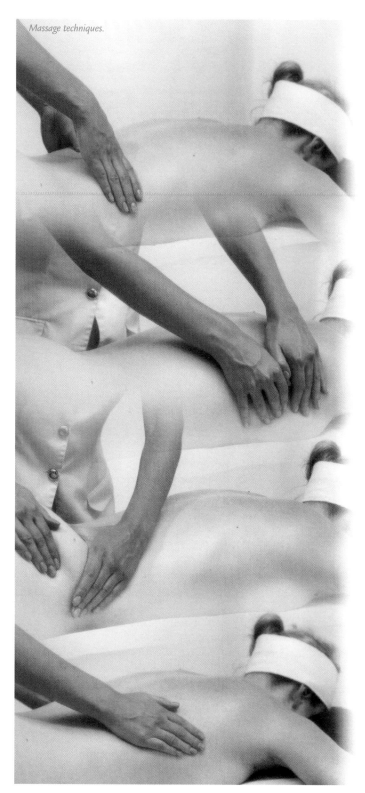

Massage techniques.

paramount importance and a professional aromatherapist will not allow any emotional or sexual involvement with the client to compromise the client's position. Vice-versa, if you feel that the client is behaving inappropriately towards you, you would be perfectly within your rights to discontinue the treatment.

- **psychology**

It is important not to become the client's counsellor. Obviously, if a client feels relaxed and comfortable with the aromatherapist, s/he may talk of their problems/thoughts but the aromatherapist must resist the temptation to get personally involved, offering judgements or advice. It is also wise to avoid topics of conversation that may cause offence or strong feelings such as money, marriage, religion or politics (especially controversial issues like abortion, capital punishment, immigration).

- **hygiene**

The aromatherapist's equipment (couch, towels, changing room, consultation room) should be kept clean at all times and the aromatherapist should also pay attention to his/her personal hygiene since they will be spending intensive periods of time in a confined space with the client.

Performing an aromatherapy massage

Each massage, just like each masseur/se and client is individual and it would thus be impossible to provide a perfect massage sequence that suits every practitioner and client. By practising the techniques described above in a suitable environment, an aromatherapist will develop their own routines adapted to each client's needs.

You now know about the practicalities and good practice that should be considered before giving a massage as well as the techniques to use in a routine. The final section explains possible allergic or adverse reactions which a practising aromatherapist will need to recognise.

REACTIONS TO TREATMENTS

When you use essential and carrier oils on the skin you are introducing a foreign substance to the body. In some cases, the body may have an adverse or allergic reaction to the oils and this may show on the skin or in other systems of the body (e.g. sneezing or asthma). This section explains the most likely and common reactions. However, it is always advisable to be aware that other adverse irritations may occur and be able to recognise them.

Skin reactions

There are three main types of skin reactions.

• cutaneous

This common skin irritation is caused by a foreign substance reacting with the mast cells of the dermis. These cells respond by producing histamine which causes an inflammation of the skin. It is a local not whole body reaction. There are four main phases:

1. a localised wheal (raised, red mark) appears on contact with the substance (a common example of this is the spotty red nettle rash, also known as a form of urticaria)

2. generalised (whole body) urticaria, inflammation and pain

3. urticaria and bronchial asthma

4. urticaria and anaphylaxis (a state of shock which occurs as a result of an antigen-antibody reaction in the cells).

• allergic/sensitivity

This is a reaction of the immune system. When it first enters the skin the foreign substance integrates with the lymphatic tissue and sensitises the T-lymphocytes. In the future, any contact with the same substance will cause the immune system to react and attack – this is an allergy. This attack usually causes skin irritations like those described above. Sometimes an allergy or hypersensitivity to a particular substance can be extremely fast and severe (nut allergies, for example, may prove fatal). Sensitising oils include benzoin, black pepper, clary sage, clove, eucalyptus, jasmine absolute, juniper, pine, rose absolute, ylang ylang.

• phototoxicity/photosensitisation

This is a very common reaction to citrus oils. The foreign substance enters the skin and fuses with the cells. When the skin is later exposed to sunlight, it will be more sensitive and may burn and/or develop melanin disorders. Photosensitising oils include bergamot, ginger, lemon, mandarin, orange, patchouli.

Non-skin reactions

All of the following may occur:
- asthma attacks
- migraines
- headaches
- severe nausea
- diarrhoea
- depression
- fatigue
- 'foggy' or 'muzzy' head.

Most of these are caused by overdosage. The strength and concentration of essential oils is such that any mistakes in dilutions or blending may cause one or several of the above. If clients are planning to buy their own oils, it is very important to explain that they need to be used diluted not neat (there are very few exceptions). In some cases it may be advisable to provide written instructions on correct use and safety implications.

AROMATHERAPY MASSAGE

How can reactions be prevented?

The first step is to take precautions by getting as much information from the client as possible and then giving them as much information as possible. This should be done in the first consultation. Any allergies to cosmetics, perfumes, toiletries, food or any family history of such allergies needs to be recorded. If any cosmetics or creams have been used on the area to be treated, especially the face and neck, the area will need to be cleansed. Any of the following will increase skin sensitivity:

- perfumes or perfumed products
- deodorants/antiperspirants
- aerobic/vigorous exercise or any activity that increases perspiration (because perspiration increases skin sensitivity).

If any cross-sensitisation or reaction occurs it should be recorded on the client card.

NB It is important to remember that –

- atopic clients (anyone who suffers from hayfever, allergic rhinitis, eczema, asthma, allergies to wool, dust or animal hair) are 13.5 times more likely to have a reaction to essential oils
- any history of melanoma or skins with large/dark moles are contra-indications for citrus oils which have been shown to increase malignancy rates.
- clients should be warned not to follow treatment with saunas, steambaths, sunbeds or beach sunbathing or waxing.

What if the aromatherapist is allergic or atopic?

The same precautions taken for clients should be taken by the aromatherapist, especially since the therapist will be spending long periods of time working with these concentrated substances. The following preventative measures should be used at all times:

- limit the amount of direct contact with neat oils.
- keep oils, both neat and diluted, away from the face and eyes. Hair should be tied up during massage but if a strand falls over the face, use the forearm to push it away from the face.
- between clients wash hands thoroughly and use an unperfumed moisture cream to protect them.
- if hands are sore or cracked do not use sensitising oils especially not absolutes which are known to cause more irritation due to the solvents used to extract them.
- limit personal use of perfumed products and cosmetics and limit exposure to household chemicals such as cleaning products/washing-up liquid (e.g. wear gloves when cleaning to protect hands). Cross-sensitisation may occur with constant exposure to perfumes or chemicals which react with the oils.

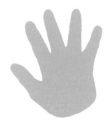

8 The holistic approach

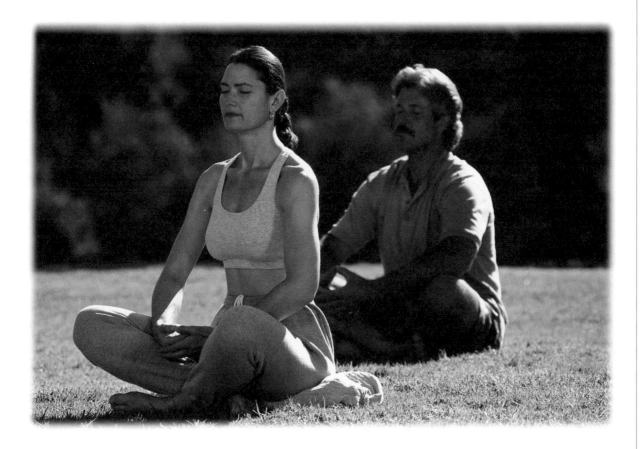

In Brief

The first section of this chapter explains the holistic approach, integral biology and why they are important for practising aromatherapists; the second explains how a holistic approach and aromatherapy can help in the treatment of hospital and hospice patients.

WHAT IS THE HOLISTIC APPROACH?

The term holistic comes from the Greek word *holos* meaning whole. The holistic approach or treatment takes into account a person's whole being, not just the physical symptoms or problems but also psychology, environment and nutrition and the effects, both positive and negative, that these can have on the body as a whole.

What is integral biology?

Integral biology is the study of our environment's effect on our physical and mental health. Everything we do in our daily lives affects our bodies. For example, an uncomfortable working environment can cause stress, tiredness and related conditions such as anxiety, depression and heart conditions. At home lack of exercise and a poor diet plus too much sedentary activity (watching TV, writing, reading, using computers) may cause similar problems.

What affects integral biology?

There are many factors that influence our integral biology. Some are negative and some positive.

Negative factors
- lack of exercise
- processed food
- chemically-treated fruit and vegetables
- lack of fresh air
- too much alcohol
- a stressful job
- bereavement or grief
- too much caffeine (tea, coffee, cola)
- lack of sleep
- financial problems
- worries about family
- worries about relationships
- too much time spent on or near electro-magnetic equipment (computers, photocopiers)
- smoky or poorly ventilated home or office
- internalising problems and worries.

Positive factors
- regular exercise
- eating fresh (preferably organic or non-chemically treated) fruit and vegetables
- a varied diet
- drinking lots of water
- taking regular breaks at work and home
- reorganising work patterns to avoid sitting or standing in the same place for several hours in a row
- getting enough sleep
- getting plenty of fresh air and making sure a window is open when someone is smoking.

How can these problems be treated by aromatherapy?

Imbalances in the external environment

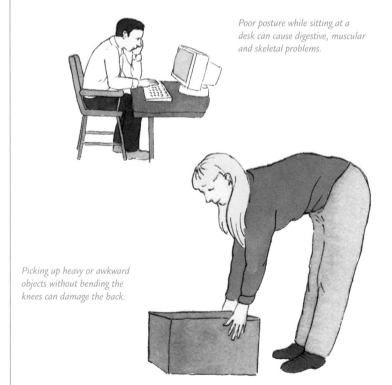

Poor posture while sitting at a desk can cause digestive, muscular and skeletal problems.

Picking up heavy or awkward objects without bending the knees can damage the back.

can cause imbalances internally. It is therefore important to take any apparently external factors into account before trying to treat physical symptoms. Poor circulation might appear to be a serious blood problem, but may be caused by lack of exercise and a diet lacking in nutrients. Aromatherapy aims to treat both the symptom and its real cause, not its probable one, in order to restore the body's equilibrium as quickly as possible.

How can an aromatherapist find out what is the real cause?

By careful questioning and discussion. When a patient comes for a massage the aromatherapist needs to find out as much as possible about the person and the problem (see Consultation Techniques in Chapter 7). Topics covered should include medical history, contra-indications to treatment, current illnesses or physical/psychological conditions, family details, type of work and working conditions, stress at work and at home, hobbies, lifestyle (i.e. sedentary, active, relaxed, stressed), diet and exercise. The aromatherapist should also look for non-verbal clues such as nervous habits and poor posture that provide information on the patient's day-to-day life. On subsequent visits the aromatherapist should check for any changes and discuss these with the patient before considering any adjustments of the oils and/or massage used.

Can aromatherapy alone cure the real cause once it is discovered?

In some cases yes. However, the aromatherapist may offer after-care advice, explaining how aromatherapy is part of the process of healing and not a miracle cure and that if the conditions that caused the problem in the first place continue then the problem will continue as well. Also, it is important to remember that aromatherapy is complementary to traditional, or allopathic, medicine rather than a replacement for it. Where appropriate it can be used at the same time as traditional medicine.

Why is a holistic approach important?

Because it treats each person individually and in the context of their own life. This enables people to help themselves to improve their health and re-establish the body's equilibrium, known as homeostasis. Furthermore, for the best therapeutic effect and the most accurate choice of oils for a treatment, all aspects of integral biology need to be considered.

You now know about the holistic approach and integral biology. The next section explains how aromatherapy may be used in a care setting such as a hospital or hospice.

THE USE OF AROMATHERAPY IN A CARE SETTING

How can aromatherapy be used in health care?

Essential oils can benefit health on physical, psychological and pharmacological levels and are thus very suitable for use in a health care environment. When ill or hospitalised, one or more of the patient's five senses may be affected. Smell is a powerful stimulant, both of the memory and the rest of the body and thus aromatherapy's combination of aromas and touch can enhance the life of a patient to great effect. With the advent of antibiotic-resistant 'superbugs' research is being undertaken using essential oils to prevent bacterial growth and assist in cases where body tissue is slow to heal.

When is it not suitable?
Using aromatherapy in any way requires communication between the medical practitioner, therapist and patient. The therapist needs to know of any contraindications to treatment and prescription medicines the patient is taking. The aromatherapist can ask the doctor to sign a letter of consent specifying the type of treatment to be performed. Some healthcare trusts decline written permission due to an increase in litigation but many doctors feel that their patients are able to take decisions about their own health.

What precautions need to be taken in this environment?
Therapists who are able to work in a care setting should be aware of and comply with any existing care plans, should keep detailed consultation forms and records and blend oils used with care and consideration. Some establishments require that oils mixed for patients are kept with other drugs, usually in a cabinet or on a locked trolley so that their use is recorded.

Is it available on the NHS?
Aromatherapy is not, at the time of writing, fully available through NHS doctors and hospitals, but many practices and private hospitals offer it as a service which patients may pay for if they wish. There are, however, several pioneering hospitals which offer aromatherapy to both patients and staff.

Is aromatherapy suitable for people with special needs or learning difficulties?
The use of essential oils in this particular setting is becoming more widespread (see for example the case study on Natalie, Chapter 10). Aromatherapy is often used in combination with specialised units such as Snoozelum rooms to enhance development and calm behaviour. Patients sometimes suffer physical problems caused by their repetitive or limited movements and the application of oils like lavender have been used to help heal and protect the skin. Benefits include improved sleep patterns and a relaxation of physical tetany (muscle spasms).

Can aromatherapy be used with the elderly?
This sector of care is enlarging dramatically as more people live on into their 80s and 90s. The traditional role of the family as carers has changed and this task is now being undertaken by professionals. Aromatherapy is particularly applicable here as many elderly people suffer the stress of bereavement, loss of their home, moving to a new area, making new friends often coupled with ill health. Loss of physical contact also plays a large part as people age and become withdrawn as a result of change. Aromatherapy works on many levels and can be used to help both physical and psychological health problems.

Can aromatherapy help the terminally ill?
Extensive research into the effects of aromatherapy in a palliative care environment (for the terminally ill or incurable) is being carried out. Essential oils are used to provide pain relief, lessen the side effects of other treatments and combat the stress experienced by patients suffering terminal illness and their families. Several programmes exist in hospitals and healthcare trusts where the importance of stress reduction, alternative pain relief and simple human

contact have been recognised. Some general hospitals are also using aromatherapy for palliative care.

Which treatments are suitable in hospital?

Essential oils may be used in a care setting in many ways:

- **massage** – limited body movement due to health problems may prevent full body massage, but massaging parts of the body that are accessible can bring about a feeling of relaxation and temporary relief from pain. Patients who cannot move around a lot particularly suffer from poor blood and lymphatic circulation and aromatherapy massage can help stimulate these. The therapist should take into account any prescribed medication and possible contra-indications when selecting oils and blending for massage. Carrier oils also need to be selected carefully as patients may have more delicate skin as a result of medication, constant wear and tear or age and some of the heavier oils may be too sticky for massage use.

- **compresses** – both hot and cold compresses may be used to ease painful joints, aching muscles or cool a fevered brow. For methods, see Chapter 4 – Application.

- **foot/hand baths** – useful for people who can't move around, yet want to experience the benefits of hydrotherapy and aromatherapy. Hot or cold water may be used and specific oils chosen depending on the patient's requirements.

- **inhalation** – the simplest method. One or two drops of oil may be put on a tissue for the patient to inhale. This method is often very useful for emotional conditions such as stress, depression or anxiety and it is also extremely portable – the patient can take the tissue wherever they go and continue inhaling the oil. Inhalation also allows the patient to choose the oils they wish to use.

- **burners/vaporisers** – care must be taken when recommending the use of burners. The use of naked flames in a care setting is prohibited so standard essential oil burners are not suitable; however electric burners can be used. These make use of a sealed electric coil under a clay or glazed ceramic bowl. The essential oil is placed in the bowl and then the burner is turned on. Oil may also be placed in the bowl with a tiny amount of water, but the vaporiser needs to be unplugged first. As with a normal burner, electric burners get very hot and need to be placed on a heatproof mat. As the coil heats, the oil vaporises into the air. Care should be taken to ensure electrical safety – no trailing wires and do not place the vaporiser near water. Manufacturers' instructions must be followed at all times. Equipment is also available in the form of nebulisers or vaporisers that use a pump to blow out a very fine mist of oil into the air. Again, manufacturers' instructions for use must be followed carefully. All electrical equipment must be subject to regular electrical safety checks in line with the insurance requirements of the care establishment. If the patient's immune system has been weakened, vaporisers are of great use with antiviral oils. Electric burners can be switched off and remain warm for hours, thereby continuing the vaporisation. Light bulb rings are also suitable if used correctly.

Are there any oils that are particularly helpful in this setting?

Patients finding themselves in a hospital, nursing/residential home, hospice, or rehabilitation unit are often stressed as a result of changes in their health and home environment. This may show physically or mentally; anxiety, depression, frustration and anger are common as are muscle and joint pains, headaches, digestive disorders, oedema and circulatory problems. Some useful oils for treating these problems are listed below and the A–Z in Chapter 5 provides information on specific oils.

Anxiety/depression/stress
Basil, benzoin, bergamot, chamomile (Roman), clary sage, cypress, frankincense, geranium, jasmine, lavender, mandarin, melissa, neroli, patchouli, petitgrain, rose, rosewood, sandalwood, sweet marjoram, vetiver, ylang ylang.

Grief/bereavement
Benzoin, chamomile (Roman), cypress, geranium, lavender, mandarin, melissa, neroli, patchouli, rose, sweet marjoram, myrrh, vetiver.

Wounds/scars/skin healing
Bergamot, chamomile (Roman and blue German), cypress, eucalyptus, frankincense, geranium, juniper, lavender, lemon, myrrh, patchouli, tea tree.

Muscular problems
Black pepper, cypress, clary sage, ginger, grapefruit, lavender, lemongrass, sweet marjoram, rosemary, thyme.

Joint problems
Benzoin, black pepper, chamomile (Roman and blue German), eucalyptus, ginger, juniper, lavender, lemon, myrrh, pine, sage, thyme, vetiver.

9 Other complementary therapies

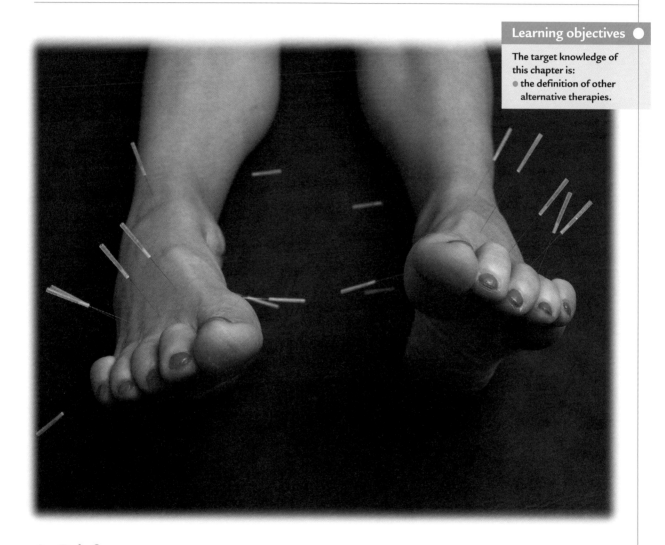

In Brief

Aromatherapy is only one of many complementary therapies.
This chapter gives a brief overview of others, many of which work
well in conjunction with essential oil treatments.

Acupuncture

An ancient Chinese therapy, now being used more and more in the West, acupuncture is the insertion of very fine needles into the skin at certain points to help relieve pain and improve the body's own healing mechanisms. The points are on meridians (energy channels). If there is a blockage in energy then a part of the body connected to that meridian may become ill or weak. The needles are thought to release the blockage and help the body to heal itself.

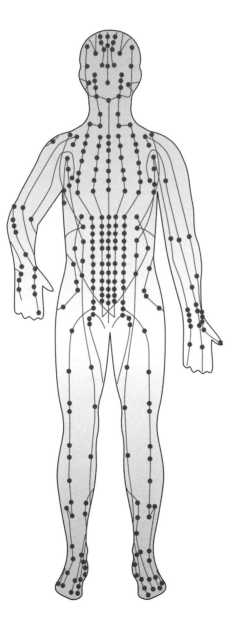

Acupuncture meridians and pressure points.

Alexander technique

The Alexander technique encourages healing and better health through better posture and awareness of how the body is used. It is especially useful for backache and headaches. It was developed by Frederick Mathias Alexander, an actor, who discovered that improving his posture stopped him losing his voice.

Bach flower remedies

Dr Edward Bach, a doctor and a practising homeopath, turned away from both traditional medicine and homeopathy believing that there was a more natural and holistic way to treat illness. He developed these 38 remedies, which are infusions of plants with water and alcohol, based on his research in the countryside. The remedies aim to treat mental and emotional problems, which often precede and cause physical symptoms.

Bowen technique

The Bowen technique, developed in Australia by Thomas A. Bowen, aims to rebalance the body holistically using gentle moves on tissues. A Bowen practitioner can feel whether muscles are stressed or tense and use the moves to release this build-up. The light rolling movements stimulate the body's energy flows. It is not a massage or a manipulation but a gentle process that encourages the body to heal itself.

Chiropractic

A chiropractor manipulates the joints of the body, specifically the spine, in order to relieve pain. It works on the basis that pain is often caused by a nerve which is not functioning properly and thus the spine, which the central nervous system runs through, is the focus of the therapy. It is especially useful for any lower back and neck pains as well as headaches.

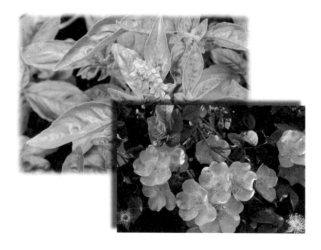

Herbalism

Herbalism is the use of plants, usually the whole plant to make herbal remedies. It is an ancient, traditional medicine – what is now considered traditional medicine only replaced it in the last three hundred years.

Homeopathy

Homeopathy treats like with like. By using minute doses of the bacteria, virus or substance which has caused the problem in the first place (i.e. cat hair in a remedy for an allergy to cat hairs) the treatment builds up the patient's resistance and immunity to the problem substance or bacteria. Homeopathic remedies and aromatherapy are rarely compatible, because one may counteract the other. Many homeopathic remedies have to be used and even stored well away from strong smells because such smells can reduce their effectiveness.

Iridology

By studying the irises (the coloured parts of the eyes) of a patient and noting any changes, iridologists can diagnose physical and psychological problems.

Kinesiology

Kinesiology is a holistic treatment that focuses on testing the muscles and energy meridians to discover and then treat the body's imbalances on all levels: chemically, energetically, physically and mentally. Using different positions and the application of pressure to the limbs, the kinesiologist can determine whether there are any energy blocks in the body and correct them through firm massage. Kinesiology is preventative and, like many complementary therapies, aims to treat the whole person.

Osteopathy

Like a chiropractor, an osteopath manipulates the joints of the body. Osteopaths work on the basis that the body's structure and function are interdependent: if the structure is

Iridology maps.

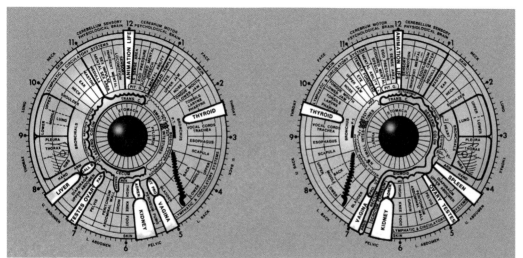

damaged in any way it will affect the function. By manipulating joints and bones they can correct structural problems which will improve the body's function. It is frequently used as a complement to aromatherapy massage.

Physiotherapy

Physiotherapy uses physical exercises, massage and the application of pressure to relieve physical pain and muscular tension. It is often used to re-educate the body in cases of major surgery, illness, or an accident.

Reflexology

This holistic therapy treats the whole person, particularly weak or ill areas, by using the feet as 'maps' of the body. On the feet there are points or zones which correspond to organs and systems of the body. By pressing on one of these points, the corresponding organ in the body is affected. For example, pressing on the tip of the big toe will cause a response in the brain and, vice versa, if there is a problem with the brain the reflexologist will recognise the symptoms of this in the big toe. This relationship, between a point on the foot and another part of the body, is known as a reflex. A trained reflexologist uses finger or thumb pressure on each of the zones to find the problem areas. He/she then applies more pressure which helps the corresponding part of the body to heal. Reflexology, unlike homeopathy, is very compatible with aromatherapy and some professionals use reflexology techniques during a massage session.

Reiki/spiritual healing

Reiki means universal life force energy in Japanese and Reiki healers act as channels for this universal energy to pass into the patient/client. By using hands in certain positions on different parts of the body, the healer is said to draw energy to the body, promoting healing, balance and relaxation.

Shiatsu

Shiatsu is a form of acupressure: the use of finger or thumb pressure on points along meridians (energy channels) to help relieve pain and encourage the body to heal itself. The pressure points are the same as those used in acupuncture.

Yoga/meditation

Both yoga and meditation have long been known to have beneficial, holistic effects and they are very useful self-help therapies. They teach the learner to have control of the body and mind. Yoga does this through physical exercise, including adopting different postures, relaxation techniques and breathing exercises. Meditation uses different focuses (such as visualisation, a candle, a mantra) to help a person find calm and a sense of their own centre. Meditation has the physiological effects of a short sleep i.e. the body goes into the healing and recharging mode it adopts when we sleep, allowing the muscles to relax and the circulation to become more efficient.

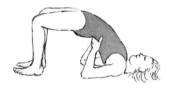

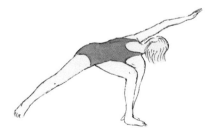

10 Case studies

Learning objectives

The target knowledge of this chapter is:
- client assessment and consultation
- the importance of keeping records
- the benefits of a series of treatments.

In Brief

Practising aromatherapists keep detailed notes about clients' treatments: their reasons for choosing aromatherapy massage, the oils used to treat the condition or problem and the reactions to and results of treatment. This final chapter provides an insight into this treatment process: it is a series of case studies which show how particular problems can be treated, the different uses and effects of oils and the possible reactions and results. *NB All names and certain details have been changed to preserve privacy. Medical history would also have been checked in detail.*

CASE STUDY 1

Client profile

Richard is a 39 year-old freelance photographer. He is HIV positive and takes combination therapy. He smokes, eats a balanced diet, does not exercise very much but gets plenty of fresh air. He loves his work, works very hard and sometimes suffers from insomnia. He chose aromatherapy for several reasons: to relax, to reduce stress and to relieve the physical symptoms of being HIV positive, one of which is very dry skin caused by taking the drugs.

Treatment plan

Four one-hour massages once a week for four weeks.

Week 1

The first massage aimed to stimulate Richard's immune system and help him to relax. The blend chosen was:
- cabbage rose (3 drops) – antidepressant and comforting
- melissa (2 drops) – antidepressant, sedative, calming
- frankincense (2 drops) – calming, reassuring, stimulates immune system.

Carrier oils: jojoba (5ml) and almond (15ml) – Richard has dry/sensitive skin and jojoba is very good for dry skin. However, it is also very thick and blending it with almond oil makes it smoother and easier to use in a massage.

Treatment summary

Richard felt a sense of well-being and comfort during the massage. It helped him to sleep better and he felt calm and relaxed for four days after the treatment.

Week 2

Richard feels more relaxed and content although he has a respiratory infection. This massage was designed to ease the respiratory infection and stimulate the immune system. The blend chosen was:
- niaouli (4 drops) – immune system stimulant, thus good for HIV clients; also good for respiratory infections
- lavender (2 drops) – cooling and anti-inflammatory, hypotensive
- lemon (2 drops) – sedative, hypotensive, anti-viral.

Carrier oil: grapeseed (20ml).

Treatment summary

Richard felt relaxed and clear-headed.

Week 3

Richard has made an effort to exercise more even though his work has kept him very busy. He is really enjoying the effects of the massages and feels very positive.

This massage focused on maintaining Richard's joyful mood, boosting his immune system and reconditioning his skin. The blend chosen was:

- patchouli (2 drops) – immuno-stimulant and good for skin
- neroli (3 drops) – cytophylactic, antidepressant, sedative
- mandarin (3 drops) – cytophylactic, uplifting, refreshing.

Carrier oil: grapeseed (20ml).

Treatment summary

Richard felt carefree, optimistic and happy after the massage and this feeling continued for a few days after the massage. He has decided to continue with massages on a regular basis.

Week 4

Though this is the last massage in this treatment plan, Richard feels that the experience has been very positive, helping him sleep and relax.

This blend aims to emphasise Richard's positive outlook and condition his skin:

- cedarwood (3 drops) – gives strength, positive, grounding
- sandalwood (3 drops) – relaxing, soothing, immuno-stimulant
- orange (3 drops) – joyful, uplifting, antidepressant.

Carrier oil: grapeseed (20ml).

Treatment summary

The smell of sandalwood had an emotionally uplifting effect on Richard, reminding him of time spent travelling in India.

Conclusion

Richard has been living with HIV for several years and takes many drugs for this. The oils were chosen to strengthen his positive outlook, stimulate his immune system and recondition his skin which has dried out as the result of taking the drugs. However, it was important to avoid over-relaxing or over-stimulating him and thus upsetting his balance since the HIV drugs already tend to relax him. The effects were positive and Richard was happy with the results.

CASE STUDY 2

Client profile

Amelia is 41 years old and has worked in the media for over 12 years. However, she is now in the process of changing careers and setting up her own garden business. She continues to work in an office in order to pay the bills and also does gardening jobs. She wants aromatherapy treatments for both emotional and physical reasons: to help her relax and accept the necessity of working in an office, to ease her tired muscles after gardening and to reduce the cellulite on her legs. She is a smoker, exercises intermittently (when gardening), sleeps well, eats a high sugar, high fat diet and does not get much fresh air when working in the office.

Treatment plan

Four one-hour massages once a week for four weeks.

Week 1

Amelia wanted to feel relaxed but also specifically asked for oils that would help her cellulite. The blend chosen was as follows:

- grapefruit (4 drops) – detoxifying, reduces fluid retention
- fennel (2 drops) – detoxifying, diuretic, reduces fluid retention
- juniper (2 drops) – stimulant, detoxifying, warming.

Carrier oils: 10ml jojoba and 10ml almond (jojoba is good for the skin and almond makes the blend smooth for use in massage).

Treatment summary

Amelia was very relaxed after the massage and happy to have done something about her cellulite. She slept very well that evening.

Week 2

Amelia wanted a relaxing massage, to help her sleep after a stressful day in the office. Rose is one of her favourite flowers and she used to wear patchouli as a perfume. Both have positive and happy associations for her. The blend chosen was:

- rose (3 drops) – soothing and sedative
- patchouli (3 drops) – sedative
- lavender (2 drops) – balancing, calming, good all-rounder, good for skin.

Carrier oils: 10ml jojoba and 10ml grapeseed (both chosen for their positive effect on the skin).

Treatment summary

Amelia really enjoyed the aromas of this massage and relaxed so much that she fell asleep. Afterwards she was very relaxed and slept well again.

Week 3

After a day of gardening, Amelia wanted a stimulating and warming massage. The blend chosen was:

- marjoram (3 drops) – warming and analgesic thus helps ease stiffness in muscles
- rosemary (3 drops) – rubefacient so stimulates circulation, eases joint pain

- lemon (2 drops) – improves circulation and removes toxins.

Carrier oils: jojoba 10ml and grapeseed 10ml.

Treatment summary

The massage had the desired effect because Amelia felt invigorated, despite being very tired.

Week 4

Amelia wanted a relaxing massage after a day spent in the office. The blend chosen, combining relaxing, calming and uplifting properties, was:

- vetiver (3 drops) – rubefacient stimulates circulation yet also tranquillising because reduces anxiety and clears mind
- frankincense (3 drops) – sedative, emotionally balancing and meditative
- mandarin (2 drops) – refreshing, uplifting and relaxing.

Carrier oils: jojoba 10ml and grapeseed 10ml.

Treatment summary

The frankincense and vetiver helped Amelia to feel relaxed and calm after a stressful day and the mandarin was an uplifting tonic.

Conclusion

Amelia needed treatment for both physical and emotional reasons and the massages helped to ease the stress and the physical effects of changing careers.

CASE STUDY 3

Client profile

Rachel is 23 years old and works in a sports centre as a lifeguard and pool attendant. She is unfulfilled in her work because she wanted promotion and hasn't been given it and although the company is now offering her a management course, Rachel is considering retraining as a firefighter. She wanted aromatherapy treatments for both emotional and physical reasons: to help her relax and solve her job indecision, to treat the spotty skin on her shoulders caused by the humid conditions at work and to relieve the headaches caused by the pool's bright lights and chemicals. Rachel gets plenty of exercise, sleeps well, drinks very little, is a non-smoker and does not eat a particularly balanced diet.

Treatment plan

Four one-hour massages once a week for four weeks.

Week 1

The first massage aimed to treat the oily, spotty skin on Rachel's shoulders and give her a boost. The blend chosen was:

- ylang ylang (3 drops) – good for oily skin, very relaxing and sedative
- lavender (3 drops) – anti-inflammatory, antidepressant, soothing qualities
- lemon (2 drops) – good for oily skin, clears toxins, refreshing, uplifting, tonic, astringent.

Carrier oils: 10ml jojoba (good for the skin because it is very similar to the skin's natural oil – sebum; also rich in vitamin E and helps to unclog pores) and 10ml almond (conditioner for skin and balances its natural oils).

Treatment summary

Rachel felt more relaxed and less anxious. She is looking forward to the next massage because she likes the feeling of calm and the lack of tension.

Week 2

Rachel's relaxed feeling continued for a couple of days after the massage but the politics at work are depressing her. She is now determined to follow a career as a firefighter and feels much more optimistic and positive about this. The skin on her shoulders is still very red. The second massage aimed to cool her skin, especially the redness on her shoulders, whilst enhancing her optimism and calm. The blend chosen was:

- myrrh (3 drops) – anti-inflammatory, cooling on skin, antiseptic, eases restlessness and calming
- frankincense (3 drops) – antiseptic, astringent, calming, meditative
- lavender (2 drops) – anti-inflammatory, soothing, antidepressant.

Carrier oils: 10ml jojoba and 10ml almond. These oils were very effective in the first massage.

Treatment summary

Rachel felt sleepy, relaxed, calm and really enjoyed the feeling of deep relaxation and peacefulness.

Week 3

Rachel is now much more refreshed, optimistic, happy and relaxed. Her muscles are more relaxed and she is not as restless. This massage will help maintain her positive attitude and continue to improve her skin condition. The oils have more woody, outdoor aromas and are therefore more uplifting. The blend chosen was:

- cedarwood (4 drops) – good for skin breakouts; strengthens mind and emotions
- juniper (1 drop) – detoxifying, relieves

worry and tension
- lavender (3 drops) – anti-inflammatory and soothing

Carrier oils: 10ml jojoba oil and 10ml almond oil.

Treatment summary

Rachel felt very content and relaxed after the massage and for once did not feel stressed at the thought of going back to work.

Week 4

Lots of positive changes have taken place in Rachel's life over the last week: the fire service have been in touch about interviewing her for a position; she is considering moving out of her parents' house to live with friends; she is eating more fruit and feeling more alert. However, she has had lots of headaches from the pool lights. In order to treat the headaches, aid concentration and cool the skin the following blend was chosen:

- eucalyptus (4 drops) – helps concentration; skin tonic
- peppermint (2 drops) – helps concentration, refreshing, relieves headaches
- lavender (2 drops) – anti-inflammatory for skin, calming

Carrier oils: 10ml jojoba and 10ml grapeseed.

Treatment summary

Rachel enjoyed the massage but felt that the blend was very cold.

Conclusion

Rachel feels more in control and more relaxed about her career choices. Overall, the massages were a success though the combination of eucalyptus with peppermint was too cooling and ginger would be a good replacement for the eucalyptus. Lavender was very effective for the skin problem.

CASE STUDY 4

Client profile

Nick is 38 years old and works in public sector housing. He had a herniated disk in his back four years ago and has regular osteopathy treatments to keep his back in good condition. His job is stressful, dealing with tenants' problems, so he wants to learn to relax body and mind, as well as relieve the general stiffness, aches and pains in his back. Nick is a smoker; he drinks very little, eats quite a healthy diet and his back pain prevents him from doing much exercise. His skin is in poor condition. The stress in his work makes him unhappy and he suffers from mild depression.

Treatment plan

Four one-hour massages once a week for four weeks.

Week 1

The aim of the first massage was to help Nick relax and ease the stiffness in his muscles. The blend chosen was:

- lavender (4 drops) – analgesic, relaxes muscle, helps CNS
- sandalwood (2 drops) – sedative, good for mild depression
- myrrh (2 drops) – calming, eases restlessness.

Carrier oils: 10ml jojoba and 10ml almond (the two oils blend well together and both are good for improving the condition of the skin).

Treatment summary

Nick felt very relaxed and calm.

Week 2

Nick commented that the massage's effects lasted well into the following week and he felt less tension at work. He was happier, refreshed and smiling. This massage concentrated on releasing emotional tension and soothing the mind. The blend chosen was:

- cypress (4 drops) – antispasmodic and sedative
- chamomile (2 drops) – anti-inflammatory and soothes nervous system
- frankincense (2 drops) – anti-inflammatory, sedative, meditative.

Carrier oils: 10ml jojoba oil and 10ml grapeseed (the jojoba is good for conditioning the skin and the grapeseed blends well and gives a smooth medium for massage).

Treatment summary

Nick felt a great sense of well-being and was very relaxed.

Week 3

Nick has had a hectic week and his muscles feel very tight. The aim of the third massage was to stimulate rather than sedate and the blend chosen was:

- ginger (4 drops) – warming, stimulant
- rosemary (2 drops) – stimulant and warming
- orange (2 drops) – uplifting and antidepressant.

Carrier oils: jojoba 10ml and grapeseed 10ml.

Treatment summary

Nick felt warm and invigorated. Though still soothing, the blend was also stimulating and refreshing.

Week 4

Nick's stressful week gave him an outbreak of dry and itchy eczema. The last massage loosened his muscles but they are now tense again. The blend chosen focused on grounding and calming Nick whilst also conditioning his skin and soothing his tense muscles:

- cedarwood (4 drops) – grounding and releases nervous tension
- patchouli (2 drops) – sedative, immuno-stimulant, good for dry skin and cytophylactic
- lavender (2 drops) – analgesic, soothes nervous system.

Carrier oils: jojoba 10ml and grapeseed 10ml.

Treatment summary

Nick felt warm, calm and less tense.

Conclusion

The massages helped Nick find a relaxed state of mind. By reducing the psychological stress, the physical tightness in his body became less of a problem.

CASE STUDY 5

Client profile

Brenda is 64 years old. She no longer works and now spends most of her time cleaning, walking and watching television. She has five children, all in their thirties and one daughter is still at home, though on the verge of moving out. Brenda is a little stressed about her daughter's imminent departure. She suffers from high blood pressure, dizzy spells, insomnia and has a stiff neck and shoulders. She is on HRT (having had a hysterectomy aged 35). She considers her days to be a bit boring. Brenda doesn't drink, smoke or eat sugar. She eats healthily and gets plenty of fresh air. She wants a series of aromatherapy massages to ease her stiffness and help her sleep.

Treatment plan

Four one-hour massages once a week for four weeks, using oils which are safe for high blood pressure (i.e. hypotensive).

Week 1

The first massage aimed to treat Brenda's stiffness whilst not over-stimulating her or aggravating her high blood pressure. It was also important to relax her in order to help her sleep. The blend chosen was:

- clary sage (4 drops) – relaxes muscles, calming, hypotensive (lowers blood pressure)
- lavender (2 drops) – soothing, calming, hypotensive, eases aches and pains
- marjoram (2 drops) – good for muscles, hypotensive, tonic for nervous system.

Carrier oils: jojoba 10ml and almond 10ml: jojoba is excellent for mature skin.

Treatment summary

Brenda felt much more relaxed and her neck and arms were less stiff. Movement was easier.

Week 2

Brenda was relaxed and less tense in her muscles after the massage. Although she requested more pressure in the next massage, this was advised against because the muscle pain may be caused by a bone not a muscle problem. This massage aimed to maintain the lightness in her muscles and neck whilst aiding sleep as well as treating the skin dryness. The blend chosen was

- melissa (3 drops) – hypotensive, sedative
- vetiver (2 drops) – sedative, aids insomnia, useful for dry, mature skins
- lavender (3 drops) – hypotensive, balancing, good for skin.

Carrier oils: jojoba 10ml and grapeseed 10ml.

Treatment summary

Brenda loved the aromas of melissa and vetiver. She became very relaxed and sleepy.

Week 3

Brenda's daughter has left home. She has had a hectic week and feels sad and at a loose end because her daughter has moved. She wants a gentle massage to lift her spirits. The massage blend was chosen for its luxurious and soothing qualities:

- neroli (4 drops) – hypotensive, eases palpitations, sedative, improves skin elasticity, relieves anxiety, luxurious and calming
- frankincense (2 drops) – meditative, emotionally reassuring
- patchouli (2 drops) – sedative, tonic, cytophylactic.

Carrier oils: jojoba 10ml and grapeseed 10ml.

Treatment summary

The massage made Brenda feel more at ease and laid-back. The blend, however, seemed rather heavy and may be improved by using one drop less patchouli and one extra drop of neroli.

Week 4

Brenda has joined a yoga class both for the physical and social benefits. She is more content and less stiff. The massage blend was chosen to enhance this positive mood, whilst conditioning her skin and not aggravating her blood pressure. The blend was:

- ylang ylang (4 drops) – hypotensive and emotionally balancing
- cabbage rose (2 drops) – antidepressant, soothing on dry maturer skin
- lavender (2 drops) – hypotensive, soothing, sedative, balancing.

Carrier oils: jojoba 10ml and grapeseed 10ml.

CASE STUDIES

Treatment summary

Brenda felt very relaxed. The oils were very suitable for reducing high blood pressure but they also reduce stress and condition the skin. However, the ylang ylang overpowered the rose and a better blend would be three drops of each to create a more balanced aroma.

Conclusion

Brenda plans to continue with massage treatments because she feels much less stiff and more relaxed. She has also joined a yoga class which helps reduce the stiffness.

CASE STUDY 6

Client profile

Peter is four years old. Normally a very active, happy and well boy, he is suffering from nasal congestion, a runny nose, sneezing, catarrh, coughing and a swollen throat. Peter drinks lots of liquids, has a balanced diet and his parents do not smoke. His parents did not wish to use conventional medicine and brought him for aromatherapy massages.

Treatment plan

Six 45-minute massages of back, neck, shoulders and face on consecutive days. Massage was preferred to inhalation since it would be difficult for Peter to use inhalations.

Massages 1 and 2

In order to release congestion and fight infection, the following blend was chosen:

- eucalyptus (1 drop) – decongestant, expectorant, good for all respiratory system problems
- tea tree (1 drop) – anti-inflammatory, antiseptic, antiviral, immuno-stimulant.

Carrier oil: 10ml evening primrose (excellent for face massage and good for dry skin) on the first occasion and 10ml peach kernel (contains vitamin E and rich in minerals) for the second massage.

Reactions to first two massages

The massages made Peter sleepy but he was still congested.

Massage 3

A different, more calming blend was chosen:

- rosewood (1 drop) – antiseptic, bactericidal, immuno-stimulant, good for respiratory infections and coughs
- scotch pine (1 drop) – antiseptic, expectorant, eases coughs and sore throat.

Carrier oil: 10ml evening primrose.

Treatment summary

Again, the massage made Peter sleepy but his cough and runny nose both seem to be improving. His mother said that he was definitely responding to the treatment and sleeping better.

Massage 4

A sedative and calming blend, with antiseptic properties, was chosen:

- scotch pine (1 drop) – antiseptic, expectorant, eases coughs and sore throats
- benzoin (1 drop) – anti-inflammatory, expectorant, eases bronchitis and coughs.

Carrier oil: 10ml peach kernel.

Treatment summary

Peter again relaxed during the treatment and seemed more lively and less congested. He slept much better that evening without coughing as much. His runny nose is getting better.

Massage 5

Sandalwood was used in this blend for its pleasant aroma and sedative qualities:

- eucalyptus (1 drop) – decongestant, expectorant, good for all problems of respiratory system
- sandalwood (1 drop) – bactericidal, antiseptic, expectorant, eases coughs, sedative.

Carrier oil: 10ml evening primrose.

Treatment summary

Peter was sleepy and relaxed during the treatment and his nose and sinuses were much better the next day.

Massage 6

This final massage aimed to maintain and strengthen the effects of the series of treatments. The blend chosen was:

- tea tree (1 drop) – anti-inflammatory, antiseptic, antiviral, immuno-stimulant
- frankincense (1 drop) – antiseptic, expectorant, calming, sedative, eases colds, flu and coughs.

Carrier oil: 10ml peach kernel.

Treatment summary

Peter is now much livelier, chattier and practically over the infection and congestion.

Conclusion

Peter's parents were very happy about his response to the treatment and especially glad that he had recovered without the use of drugs or tablets. Peter was back to his normal active self and his parents were so pleased by the response that they brought their elder son for treatment.

CASE STUDY 7

Client profile

Ian is 58 years old and suffers from muscular aches and pains and sciatic nerve problems. He works in television and thus spends long periods standing up which aggravates the pain. He is a non-smoker and eats a varied diet. He does not drink very much alcohol or very much fluid and does not get a lot of exercise. He is not on any medication. He wants to relieve his muscular aches and pains and improve his general well-being.

Treatment plan

Four full body massages once a week for four weeks.

Week 1

Ian is tall and well-built and has very hairy skin. A proportionately larger amount of base oil was thus prepared.

The first massage focused on relaxing Ian and stimulating yet soothing his aching muscles. The blend chosen for the body was:

- lavender (3 drops) – analgesic, calming, balancing, good for muscular aches and pains
- rosemary (3 drops) – tonic, poor circulation, stimulant, good for muscular aches and pains.

Carrier oils: 10ml calendula and 10ml St. John's Wort (this is a synergetic blend which complements the essential oils chosen; it is also anti-inflammatory and eases bruises and aches) plus 7.5ml sweet almond.

The blend chosen for the face was:

- neroli (1 drop) – nervous system stimulant, tonic, good for mature skin, astringent.

Carrier oil: 5ml sweet almond.

Treatment summary
Ian was so relaxed that he slept through the second half of the massage. He awoke feeling very refreshed and calm.

Week 2
The blend chosen focused on reducing muscle tension and pain as well as relaxing the body in general. The oils used for the body were:

- benzoin (3 drops) – anti-inflammatory, sedative, relieves tension, improves circulation
- scotch pine (3 drops) – stimulant, good for poor circulation, aches and pains, stress.

Carrier oils: 5ml each calendula and St. John's Wort, 15ml coconut (a light oil and a good emollient for skin and hair).

The blend chosen for the face was:

- lemon (2 drops) – antispasmodic, diuretic, good for poor circulation.

Carrier oil: 5ml sweet almond.

Treatment summary
Ian again relaxed and fell asleep. Coconut oil proved to be much better for a hairier body. Ian commented on how relaxed he felt and how much energy he had after the massage.

Week 3
This massage continued the treatment of the first two weeks: stimulating the muscles to relieve tension whilst sedating the mind to encourage relaxation. It also aimed to ease Ian's nasal congestion. The oils chosen for the body were

- lavender (3 drops) – analgesic, calming, sedative, tonic, stimulates circulation
- black pepper (3 drops) – analgesic, stimulates circulation, warming (thus easing aches and pains).

Carrier oils: 5ml each calendula and St. John's Wort, 15ml coconut.

The blend chosen for the face was:

- sandalwood (1 drop) – sedative, expectorant, tonic, relieves stress.

Carrier oil: 5ml peach kernel (rich in vitamin E thus good for the skin).

Treatment summary
Ian fell asleep and woke feeling very relaxed. He continued to feel the benefit of the massage for the rest of the week.

Week 4
Ian's congestion seems to be easing and he feels very relaxed, having slept well all week. The oils chosen for the body aimed to maintain this relaxation:

- rosemary (3 drops) – stimulant, poor circulation, aches and pains, exhaustion, stress
- ginger (3 drops) – analgesic, stimulant, aches and pains, relieves tiredness and exhaustion.

Carrier oils: 5ml each calendula and St. John's Wort, 15ml coconut.

The blend chosen for the face was:

- bergamot (1 drop) – uplifting, stimulant, tonic, relieves stress and anxiety.

Carrier oil: 5ml sweet almond.

Treatment summary
Ian relaxed and slept. His muscles felt firmer but less tense.

Conclusion
The pain in Ian's neck, shoulder and leg had been greatly reduced and the massages had also helped his sleeping patterns. He had taken up the suggestion of increasing his fluid intake and taking regular exercise and felt much better. Ian was pleasantly surprised by the thoroughness of the whole aromatherapy massage and consultation and felt that he would continue with lots of the suggestions made to improve his health and fitness.

CASE STUDY 8

Client profile

Natalie is 33 years old. She was brain-damaged at birth and registered blind (95% loss of sight). She lives in a residential home with five adults plus a live-in residential worker. She has an active lifestyle, eats a varied diet (with a tendency to put on weight), doesn't smoke or drink and is very calm and relaxed. Her posture is poor and she drinks six to eight large cups of strong black coffee every day. She has come for aromatherapy massage for several reasons: to stimulate her circulation, help eliminate chronic body odour and halitosis and to improve her digestion and ease her constipation.

Treatment plan

Four full body massages once a week for four weeks.

Week 1

The first massage aimed to gently introduce Natalie to aromatherapy treatment whilst stimulating her circulation and digestion. The blend of oils chosen was:

- carrot seed (3 drops) – carminative, diuretic, vasodilatory, depurative
- black pepper (3 drops) – carminative, depurative, stimulant, tonic.

Carrier oils: 15ml sweet almond (rich in vitamins and minerals and suitable for all skin types), 10ml peach kernel (contains vitamin E, good for dehydrated skins).

The blend chosen for the face was:

- cabbage rose (1 drop) – depurative, tonic, astringent, relaxing, sedative.

Carrier oil: 5ml jojoba (resembles skin's natural oils and rich in vitamin E).

Treatment summary

Though apprehensive at first, Natalie was very relaxed by the end of the treatment and looking forward to the next massage. It was suggested that Natalie should replace her coffee intake with water and fruit juices and try to eat more fibre.

Week 2

Natalie was very excited about her second massage. She has made an effort to drink less coffee and more juice. Her constipation has not been so chronic and her body odour has lessened. The blend of oils chosen again concentrated on aiding digestion and stimulating the circulation:

- black pepper (3 drops) – carminative, depurative, stimulant, tonic
- juniper (3 drops) – carminative, diuretic, sedative.

Carrier oils: 15ml sweet almond, 10ml peach kernel.

The blend chosen for the face was:

- patchouli (1 drop) – antidepressant, diuretic, sedative, tonic.

Carrier oil: 5ml jojoba.

Treatment summary

Natalie was much more relaxed and felt less congested around the colon. She has promised to keep reducing her coffee intake.

Week 3

Again, Natalie was very excited about her treatment. Her key worker noted that she had been less constipated and that her body odour and halitosis had improved. The blend of oils chosen was:

- marjoram (3 drops) – antispasmodic, tonic, relaxing, sedative, good for digestive system
- grapefruit (3 drops) – diuretic, stimulant, uplifting, refreshing.

Carrier oils: 15ml sweet almond, 10mls calendula (anti-inflammatory and good for aches, pains and bruises).

The blend chosen for the face was:
- mandarin (1 drop) – carminative, diuretic, sedative, tonic, refreshing.

Carrier oil: 5ml jojoba.

Treatment summary
Natalie was relaxed and happy.

Week 4
Natalie was a little tired but very excited. Her key worker mentioned that she was less constipated and generally contented. Her weight was steady but she still had a slight body odour. The blend of oils chosen was:
- mandarin (3 drops) – carminative, diuretic, sedative, tonic, refreshing
- grapefruit (3 drops) – diuretic, stimulant, uplifting, refreshing.

Carrier oils: 10mls calendula and 15ml peach kernel.

The blend chosen for the face was:
- cabbage rose (1 drop) – depurative, tonic, astringent, relaxing, sedative.

Carrier oil: 5ml peach kernel.

Treatment summary
Natalie was very relaxed and slept through most of the massage. When she woke she was excited and happy.

Conclusion
Natalie's constipation has improved and she has made a real effort to drink more water and less coffee. Her body odour was reduced greatly as was her bad breath. She was also very serene and content after the massages and felt very happy thanks to the treatments.

Bibliography

- Arnould-Taylor, WE, *Aromatherapy for the Whole Person* (Leckhampton: Stanley Thornes, 1981)

- Davis, Patricia, *Aromatherapy: an A-Z* (Saffron Walden: C.W.Daniel, 1999)

- Lawless, Julia, *The Encyclopaedia of Essential Oils* (Shaftesbury: Element, 1992; reprinted 2000)

- Maxwell-Hudson, Clare, *The Complete Book of Massage* (London: Dorling Kindersley, 1988)

- Price, Shirley, *The Aromatherapy Workbook* (London: Thorsons, 1998)

- Price, Shirley and Len, *Aromatherapy for Health Professionals* (Edinburgh: Churchill Livingstone, 1995)

- Room, Adrian (Ed), *Brewer's Dictionary of Phrase and Fable*, 15th edition (London: Cassell, 1997)

Glossary

Absolute: thick liquid made from blending concrete with alcohol, then removing alcohol by evaporation

Acupuncture: Chinese technique involving the insertion of needles into energy points of the body

Adulterate: change the purity (and thus the effectiveness) of an essential oil by various methods of dilution and substitution

Aromatherapy: the use of essential oils and plant essences in therapeutic treatments

Aromatic: having a smell, or fragrance

Atom: the tiniest particle of matter

Avicenna: credited with developing/ inventing distillation technique for extracting oils

Ayurvedic medicine: traditional Indian herbal medicine

Carrier oil: an oil from a plant, flower, nut or seed, used in blend with essential oils for treatments. Carrier can also be creams, gels or shampoos

Chemotype: a plant that is botanically identical to another (two rose bushes for example) but chemically different because it has been grown in different conditions (different geographical place, altitude, climate, cultivation)

Concrete: waxy residue containing plant essence that is obtained through solvent extraction

Desquamation: the flaking-off of dead skin cells

Elasticity: the ability to stretch

Element: the purest state of a chemical component

Essence: a plant's oil (not yet extracted or extracted by expression)

Essential oil: a plant's essence (that has been extracted by distillation)

Gattefossé, René Maurice: French scientist who reintroduced the use of essential oils in complementary therapy to the Western world and invented the term 'aromathérapie'

Herbal: a book on the subject of herb/plant properties, uses and benefits (common in 18th and 19th centuries)

Hippocrates: 'father of medicine'; greatly added to and developed knowledge and use of plants and herbs in medical remedies

Holistic: addressing the whole, not just a part

Hydrocarbon: a molecule made of hydrogen and carbon atoms

Hydrolat: aromatic or scented water, often the by-product of distillation

Inorganic: non-living

Integral: concerning the whole, not just a part

Maury, Marguerite: Austrian biochemist who brought aromatherapy to Britain

Molecule: a group of atoms joined together

'Nature-identical': synthetic oils that contain some organic molecules from cheap essential oils

Organic: living

Oxygenated compound: a molecule made of hydrogen, carbon and oxygen atoms

Percolation: distillation process that uses steam but pushes steam down through the plant material instead of up

Pharmacological: a chemical effect

Photosynthesis: the process by which a plant captures the energy of the sun, via a pigment in its leaves called chlorophyll, and uses it to convert carbon dioxide into organic substances

Phototoxicity: skin is sensitive to and possibly damaged by sunlight

Physiological: a physical effect

Pomade: fatty solid containing plant essence that is obtained through enfleurage

Psychological: an effect on the mind

Shiatsu: Chinese technique using the same energy points as acupuncture but applying finger and thumb pressure to them instead of using needles

Solvent extraction: use of a chemical substance to extract plant essence

Stable: will not evaporate in air

Still: the equipment used to extract plant essences by distillation: consists of vessel for holding plant material, pipes to transfer steam, condenser, heat source

Synergy: how all the different molecules of an oil combine and work together as a whole oil, producing different effects to those of each molecule group used individually

Trace element: a tiny amount of an element

Valnet, Jean: French doctor who continued the work of Gattefossé

Volatile: will evaporate in air